THE ESSENTIAL GUIDE
TO CANNABIS FOR WOMEN

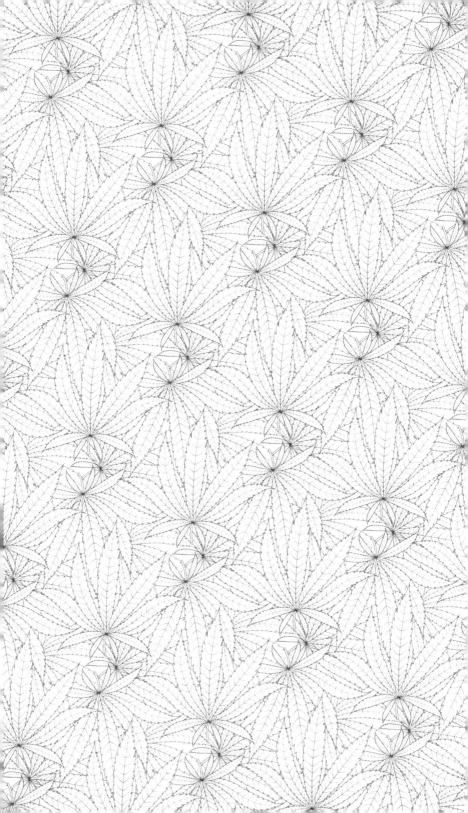

The ESSENTIAL GUIDE TO CANNABIS *for* Women

How to Buy, Use, and Enjoy Cannabis for Recreation and Wellness

OLIVIA ALEXANDER

ROCKRIDGE
PRESS

For general information on our other products and services or to obtain technical support, please contact our Customer Care Department within the United States at (866) 744-2665, or outside the United States at (510) 253-0500.

Rockridge Press publishes its books in a variety of electronic and print formats. Some content that appears in print may not be available in electronic books, and vice versa.

Interior and Cover Designer: Scott Wooledge
Art Producer: Alyssa Williams
Editor: Nora Spiegel
Production Manager: Riley Hoffman

All illustrations used under license from Shutterstock.com.
Author photo courtesy of Molly Pan Photography.

Paperback ISBN: 978-1-63807-705-3
eBook ISBN: 978-1-63807-540-0
R0

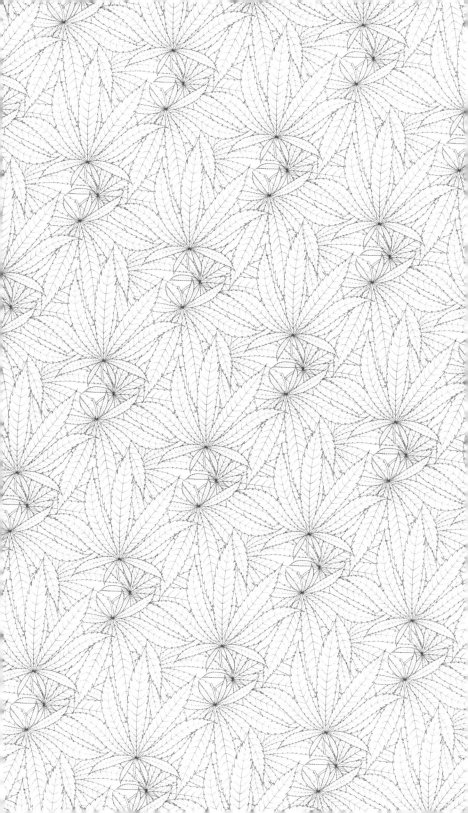

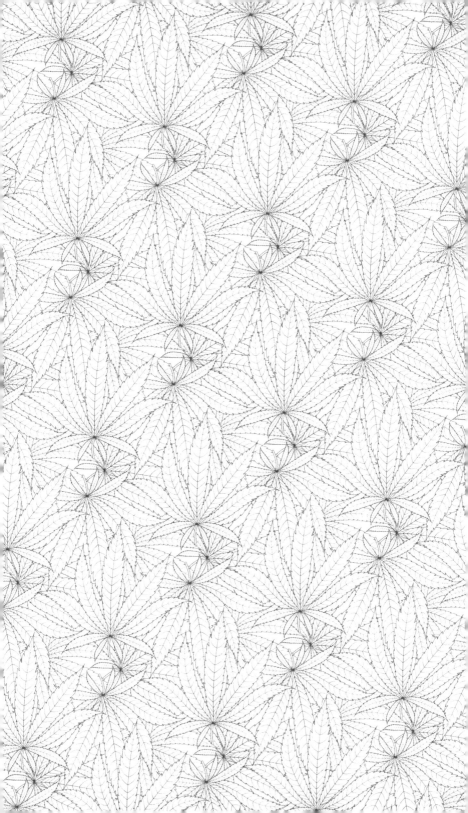

CONTENTS

INTRODUCTION

THE LIGHTER FLICKED, THE FLAME DANCED, I FELT THE smoke fill my lungs as I inhaled. I exhaled. And then I realized that everything I had been taught about this plant was based on fear and, perhaps, lies. Fear had kept me from understanding a gentle, giving plant that offered a vast spectrum of uses.

Before you experience cannabis for yourself, the idea can seem scary or unapproachable. That's okay. For those who are new to the plant, it's normal to not know where to start. Maybe you've tried cannabis with friends, but have never bought it yourself. Once you become comfortable exploring and testing out different kinds of cannabis, you can discover a world of healing and new experiences. For me, that first puff put an end to my years-long battle with insomnia. That same night, for the first time in as long as I could remember, I slept the deep sleep I was always needing but could never find.

Over the years, I further developed my relationship with cannabis. I would lean on it when my body ached, and I would always have it available when I was on my period. Cannabis would transform my ability to manage my bipolar symptoms. I've spent over 15 years working in the cannabis trade, beginning long before it was legalized, and today in the legal cannabis market in California. I started behind the counter of a dispensary, where I came to understand how many people use cannabis not just for getting high but for their own wellness. I have grown, extracted, and made products with cannabis. And along the way I've developed a unique understanding of the relationship between cannabis and women, who are one of the largest growing demographics of cannabis consumers, but whose needs and lifestyle don't always fit the mold of the stereotypical stoner.

As a young woman working with cannabis products, I quickly realized that not only were there very few of us in the industry, there were very few cannabis products made for women specifically. In 2015, after spending years in the trenches, I started my own company, Kush Queen, to create products for everyone who didn't identify with the typical stoner experience. Today our company produces over 80 award-winning products in-house, for women, by women. Unlike many recreation-focused brands, we center on the female consumer and cannabis experience, and have invested heavily in cannabis education, innovation in technology and formulas, and wellness approaches to mental health and pain.

From stress, anxiety, and menopause to menstrual cycles, women love to use cannabis to manage their wellness and improve their lives. Whether you're new to this idea or an old pro looking to expand your knowledge, this book will help you chart the course of your cannabis journey. We'll begin with cannabis 101, exploring the history of this remarkable plant, digging into the science behind cannabis and the endocannabinoid system, and demystifying some myths about cannabis and its use. Then, in part 2, we'll explore practical applications of cannabis use for mental health, fitness, aging, and in the bedroom (for both sleep and sex). Empowered with all that knowledge, you'll be ready to create cannabis products of your own, using some favorite family recipes I'll share with you in part 3.

Cannabis is so much more than a plant; its story is intertwined with social justice issues and with medicine. A wellness tool for some, and a way to have fun for others, cannabis intersects with many problems that currently plague millions of Americans. In 1996, California (the fifth-largest economy in the world) legalized medical cannabis in the state. Since then, state by state, we have seen laws reversed and significant progress made, and this has all been driven by the will of voters at the ballot box. A 2021 survey by the Pew Research Center shows that over 90 percent of Americans believe cannabis should be legal in some form. As we enter the second decade of the 21st century, our country's attitude towards cannabis is at a significant crossroads, with many health epidemics and the stresses of a global pandemic driving millions of people to cannabis for the first time. It's an incredible time in the world of cannabis. I hope, like me, you're excited to see where cannabis use and culture is headed in the coming years.

One final note before we begin: You'll notice that I always refer to the plant as cannabis, not marijuana. "Cannabis" is the correct scientific term. More on this in chapter 1 (see page 4).

Now take a deep breath and let go of all preconceived notions about cannabis. Remember, it's just a plant.

Although I will be talking about how cannabis can help with mental health and pain management, among other wellness topics, please remember this book is not intended to act as a substitute for professional medical care or licensed therapeutic guidance. Consult your doctor or a licensed professional regarding important medical and mental healthcare decisions.

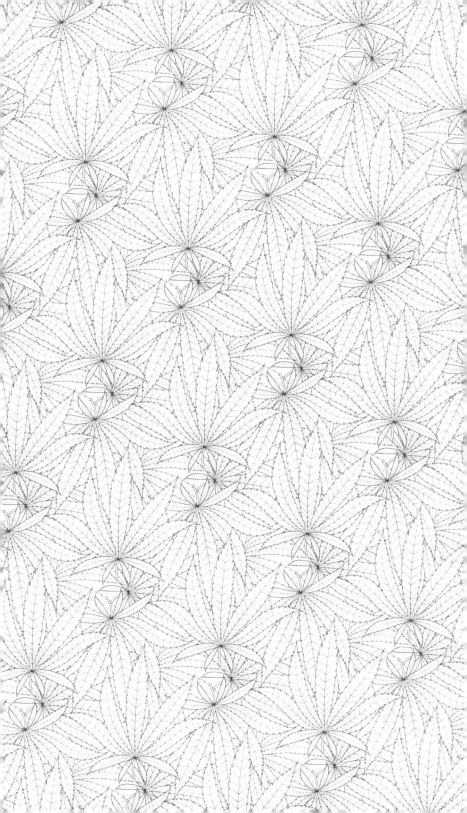

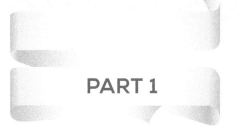

PART 1

CANNABIS 101

I HOPE THAT SOME ALCHEMICAL mixture of curiosity and desire brought you to these pages to absorb, learn, and potentially enhance your life with cannabis, even though it's perhaps very unfamiliar to you. In this section of the book, we will begin by learning about every important facet of this beautiful plant. We'll shine a light on how cannabis may benefit you, as it has already benefited others for many thousands of years. I'll also share some advice that will be essential for the experiences ahead of you. Although you may be new to cannabis, you'll soon be on your way to deep, lasting knowledge and appreciation.

CHAPTER 1

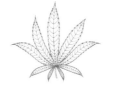

Cannabis, Demystified

CANNABIS IS A BEAUTIFUL, HEALING PLANT provided to us by nature. Due to its complicated history, it may seem a scary or intimidating substance. But as someone who's been working in cannabis for over 15 years, I'm here to help you gain a greater understanding of this plant, how it works with our bodies to provide relief, and how it can enhance our daily life in unexpected ways. Once you gain some basic knowledge, you will understand the wonder and power this plant can bring.

An All-Too-Brief (Yet Decidedly Illuminating) History of Cannabis

Early on in my exploration and education, I was amazed to learn that cannabis has been used in cultures all over the world, for many thousands of years. There is evidence that hemp was cultivated in Japan all the way back to at least 8000 BCE. That's ten thousand years ago! But since we're mentioning hemp in history, let's quickly break down the distinction between hemp and cannabis.

Actually, the two are the *exact same species of plant*. So, how are they different? For starters, hemp was originally cultivated for its fibrous stalks, not for its flowers (which contain the mood-affecting chemicals the plant's known for). Ancient cultures in Asia used this fiber to create rope and clothing. The current definition of hemp in the United States comes from the Farm Bill of 2018, according to which hemp is cannabis that contains less than 0.3 percent of the chemical tetrahydrocannabinol (THC) by dry weight. (THC is the main active mood-affecting chemical in cannabis.)

In terms of its use, researchers have discovered indications that cannabis was being smoked for religious purposes in China as far back as 2500 BCE. Convincing evidence also shows that around 8th century BCE, during the Kingdom of Judah, cannabis was being used in Tel Arad for ritualistic purposes. Fast-forward to the turn of the millennium, and we find cannabis spreading around the world, being used not only as a powerful medicine but as a recreational drug. Hashish, or cannabis resin, started to become a commodity and was used and traded in places like Iraq and Africa. In 1798, when Napoleon and his army invaded Egypt, the troops discovered the pleasures of hashish and brought it back home with them.

In the United States, before the early 20th century, cannabis and hemp were not only legally unrestricted in their uses but widely employed in the medical industry for the powerful compounds the plant contained. Then the 1906 Pure Food and Drug Act labeled cannabis as a dangerous drug and restricted its sale. In 1937, the Marihuana Tax Act made cannabis use illegal for non-medical purposes. A main proponent of this prohibition was the newspaper baron and paper producer, William Randolph Hearst. He was quoted saying, *"Users of marijuana become STIMULATED as they inhale the drug and are LIKELY TO DO ANYTHING. Most crimes of violence in this section, especially in country districts, are laid to users of that drug."*

This absurd claim was the beginning of what would be known as the "reefer madness" depiction of cannabis (*Reefer Madness* is the title of an infamous 1936 anticannabis short film). During this time, cannabis use became heavily racialized and vilified in the media. Prohibitionists adopted the exotic-sounding term "marijuana" to emphasize the plant's foreignness and play into xenophobic and racist fears among white Americans. Access was completely shut down, even for true medical use, and production and consumption were driven underground, effectively creating the black market we still know today. Because of this history, the word "marijuana" still carries a racist stigma.

It would take many decades before any progress was made in establishing a more reasoned public opinion of cannabis use. Presidents Nixon, Reagan, and Bush all waged a failed war on drugs, with cannabis as a rationale for imprisoning millions of people (disproportionately Black and Hispanic people). According to the ACLU, the same usage rates are reported across all races, but Black people are 3.64 times more likely than white people to be arrested for cannabis possession.

In 1976, Robert Randall won a court case ruling that his cannabis use was a medical necessity. Subsequently, 35 US states enacted legislation recognizing the medicinal value of cannabis. In the 1980s, the non-profit Alliance for Cannabis Therapeutics (ACT) paved the way for Proposition 215, which was passed in California in 1996. That legislation effectively restarted the medical cannabis industry, paving the way for progress not only in America but around the world, turning criminals into healers and outlaws into entrepreneurs.

As I write this, 19 states and Washington, DC, allow legal recreational cannabis use, and 37 states, plus DC, allow some form of medical use. Americans of all colors, ages, races, and walks of life believe in their right to use cannabis. The times are not just changing, they have changed.

FIVE INFLUENTIAL WOMEN IN CANNABIS HISTORY

All of the cannabis we consume grows from botanically female plants, so perhaps it's no coincidence that women have championed its use for thousands of years. Women have not only used cannabis for treating menstrual pain and other complaints; they've fought the good fight to keep the plant available. Here are five of the most influential women in cannabis history.

Hatshepsut
Egyptian Pharaoh, reigned 1479–1458 BCE

Hatshepsut, one of the few female Egyptian pharaohs, was known to use hemp to manage painful menstrual symptoms. This made her not just a trailblazer as an ambitious and successful ruler but a true cannabis pioneer. Her reign only ended when she died.

Queen Victoria
British monarch, 1819–1901

Queen Victoria ruled the United Kingdom in a strictly conservative time; however, she had one wildly progressive tool for managing her menstrual pain: cannabis. In his 2014 book *Drugged: The Science and Culture behind Psychotropic Drugs*, author Richard J. Miller notes, "Even Queen Victoria was prescribed a tincture of cannabis. It is believed she was amused (perhaps very amused)."

Alice B. Toklas
Author, 1877–1967

Pot brownies are one of the most, if not *the* most, famous cannabis edibles. The use of edibles in religion and for pleasure has been around for centuries. But there was no popularized recipe for modern users until a queer woman published instructions for "Hashish

Fudge." And just like that, *The Alice B. Toklas Cookbook* (1954) gave the iconic stoner treat its start—and even immortalized Toklas's last name in pot culture. Ever wonder where the term "toke" came from?

Margaret Mead
Academic, 1901–1978
An American cultural anthropologist and outspoken cannabis advocate, in 1969, Margaret Mead testified to the US Senate that anyone over the age of 16 should be able to legally use cannabis. In the speech, Mead said that keeping cannabis illegal was "a new form of tyranny by the old over the young." She continued to advocate for cannabis as a therapeutic and against the war on drugs for the next decade.

"Brownie" Mary Jane Rathbun
Activist, 1922–1999
Twenty years after Toklas's hit cookbook was published, Mary Jane Rathbun (yes, her name is actually Mary Jane!) was working at a San Francisco IHOP, perfecting her own pot brownie recipe in her free time. Rathbun soon began selling her "magically delicious" brownies on the streets of San Francisco's gay Castro district, quickly gaining notoriety in the city. A few years into her sales, Rathbun began to notice the health benefits of her cannabis-infused pastries for her chronically ill customers. Despite many run-ins with the law, Rathbun kept selling brownies but became more involved as an advocate and an ally to the cannabis and LGBTQ+ community. In 1991, her work with gay cannabis advocate Dennis Peron came to fruition when Prop P was passed with 80 percent of the San Francisco vote. A year later, Peron and Rathbun opened the first public dispensary in the nation, the San Francisco Cannabis Buyers Club.

How Cannabis Works in Harmony with Our Bodies

The first night I ever smoked cannabis, what surprised me most was the sleep that came after the effects wore off. It was by far the deepest, most restful sleep I'd ever had. I had suffered from insomnia since I was a young child, so this revelation was truly eye-opening (though first it was blissfully eye-closing). I wondered how this drug I'd been taught to fear could do so much good. It wouldn't be until many years later that I finally came to understand how cannabis works synergistically with our bodies, due to a critically important and understudied system in the body called the endocannabinoid system, or ECS.

The ECS is a network of chemical signals and receptors in our brain and elsewhere that respond to those signals. The ECS influences the central nervous system, which regulates our most important bodily functions: sleep, mood, appetite, pain sensation, and memory. It helps us maintain physiological, emotional, and cognitive stability. Simply put, the ECS is involved in creating homeostasis—balance and harmony—within the body. Our body is full of ECS receptors that react to cannabinoids, naturally occurring compounds produced in our body and found in the cannabis plant. This creates the myriad of effects and benefits we get from ingesting cannabis and its components. Our skin and the pain pathway of our spine, for example, have ECS receptors, and these receptors are activated by cannabinoids that come from cannabis or are produced within our own body.

Scientists have discovered over 113 cannabinoids and are discovering new ones every day. Some of the most well-known examples are tetrahydrocannabinol (THC) and cannabidiol (CBD). When these cannabinoids are ingested or put onto our skin, they interact with the ECS. Cannabinoids are known to help with sleep, mood, appetite, pain, inflammation, and nausea. Some can even boost energy, reduce appetite, and enhance mental clarity and focus.

Cannabis is an incredibly powerful plant, not only because of the myriad of compounds it creates but also because of how intertwined our endocannabinoid system is with our health. The ECS is truly a power player when it comes to wellness, because it doesn't just work in harmony with our body, it *creates* harmony within our body.

Cannabis Compounds to Know (and Love)

Cannabis is a plant, but the compounds of focus within the plant are called *cannabinoids*. There are over a hundred known naturally occurring cannabinoids, and more are being discovered constantly. Some are psychoactive (which means they affect your mood and perception), while others are nonpsychoactive. We can also describe these qualities as impairing and nonimpairing, or euphoric and noneuphoric. Along with the popular cannabinoids that most know of, THC and CBD, there are also many lesser-known "minor" cannabinoids contained within the plant that are becoming more studied and more used. Minor cannabinoids are generally less abundant but no less valuable; THCV (tetrahydrocannabivarin), CBG (cannabigerol), and CBN (cannabinol) are a few important examples we'll be mentioning in this book. All of these compounds interact with our endocannabinoid system (a.k.a. the ECS) to create effects and benefits within our bodies. The range of cannabis compounds has a myriad of benefits, from regulating sleep, mood, and appetite to managing pain, so let's take a closer look at a few star players.

THC

Tetrahydrocannabinol, or THC, is the most popular cannabis compound. When it comes to consuming cannabis, this is what all the fuss is about. Why? Because THC is the psychoactive molecule that gets you high. But even though the psychoactive properties get THC its hype, the compound has many different applications and uses. THC is a powerful anti-inflammatory molecule that can be used to treat pain, alter mood, relieve stress, and calm anxiety. THC mimics the neurotransmitter anandamide, a chemical messenger that's produced in the brain. So THC changes how your brain operates, in subtle but powerful ways. According to the National Institute on Drug Abuse, and my personal research, THC can affect our pleasure, memory, thinking, concentration, movement, coordination, and sensory and time perception. Thus, it is not recommended to drive or operate heavy machinery while using THC. Negative effects of THC are often experienced with overuse and include headaches, dizziness, drowsiness, and fatigue.

It's undeniable that certain aspects of THC have been given a bad rap, but that's only one side of the molecule's stigmatized qualities. THC shows wondrous potential not just for supporting wellness but for treating very serious diseases like eating disorders, PTSD, epilepsy, and depression. Currently, only synthetic versions of THC are approved by the Food and Drug Administration. They can produce harsh, sometimes frightening and unpleasant effects that are less likely with plant-sourced THC.

CBD

If the mainstreaming of cannabis was a large door we had to open, CBD (cannabidiol) was the key that unlocked it. This molecule wasn't front and center until recently but is now considered to be a major cannabinoid. Discovered in 1940, CBD is now a mainstream molecule, found in nearly every cannabis product and, somewhat unfortunately, touted as a cure-all by many.

Unlike THC, CBD is a non-impairing molecule, so it doesn't get you high. It can be derived from the cannabis plant or a hemp plant (which, as we mentioned, is a plant with low amounts of THC). CBD has undeniably helped normalize cannabis use. Perhaps the most exciting scientific evidence relating to the use of CBD is in managing treatment-resistant disorders around childhood epilepsy, like Dravet syndrome and Lennox-Gastaut syndrome (LGS). The seizure medication Epidiolex is the only drug containing CBD that's regulated by the Food and Drug Administration.

After the mainstreaming of CBD, we saw this chemical get infused into *everything*. Due to the popularity of CBD and its unregulated status, there was a complete free-for-all, with companies producing inaccurately dosed products and making endless false claims. Many companies have received notices from the FDA for their attempts at claiming CBD as a panacea. CBD can help with inflammation, but it is certainly not able to cure any and every disease or symptom. These bad actors have cast a great shadow of doubt over an incredibly benevolent molecule. But anecdotal evidence shows CBD to have incredible promise. Its popularity is in part due to its efficacy in changing so many people's lives and the rapid evolution its reputation has undergone to become a universally recognized wellness product.

While CBD refers to the molecule itself, there are several different ways CBD can be presented and added to products. We'll be referring to these options throughout this book:

Full-Spectrum CBD. Also called whole-plant CBD, this term indicates a full, unadulterated cannabinoid profile. This means the plant is extracted and the entire cannabinoid and terpene content is preserved (terpenes are another class of chemicals that we'll talk more about in a bit). This is the best option for CBD products, since we know that cannabinoids and terpenes all work better together (that's called the "entourage effect," and we'll talk more about that, too). Know that full-spectrum products do contain THC and so can produce a mildly sedative effect that can be strong for some new users.

Broad-Spectrum CBD. This designation means that a product contains other cannabinoids, but the contents have gone through a process that removes all or nearly all of the THC content. Due to drug testing and international hemp laws, we see a large number of products on the market using naturally occurring cannabinoid profiles with the THC removed or brought down to a nondetectable level.

CBD Isolate. A CBD isolate product appears like a white crystalline powder and generally tests at 99 percent CBD or higher. There are generally no other cannabinoids present in CBD isolate. This is the lowest-cost option when it comes to CBD products and is best for people who are very strictly drug tested. Be aware that CBD isolate can be synthetic and depending on your needs may be an inferior option compared to a full-spectrum plant extract.

In chapter 2, we'll dive deeper into CBD and examine the facts and fiction behind some of the claims made about it.

YOUR THC VS. CBD CHEAT SHEET

THC	CBD
Impairing/euphoric (it gets you high)	Nonimpairing/noneuphoric (doesn't get you high)
Relaxant	Neuroprotectant (protects nerve cells)
Great for sleep	Antioxidant
Can cause anxiety	Used to combat anxiety
Great for analgesic pain relief	Anti-inflammatory properties
Great for treating muscular spasticity	Great for alleviating IBS symptoms
Used for nausea	Great for many mental disorders

Terpenes

You may say to yourself when opening a fresh jar of cannabis that it smells like something familiar. Orange, lavender, black pepper, lemon, even complex earthy and spicy notes are very common in cannabis, often all layered on top of each other in a complex bouquet unlike any other plant's aroma. Cannabis contains naturally occurring aromatic compounds called terpenes, which are also found in abundance in citrus trees, fragrant herbs like sage, lavender, and thyme, and many other familiar plants. Along with influencing the smell and taste of cannabis, terpenes are a powerful and underappreciated modulator of the cannabis plant's effects.

Terpenes are important to the experience of using cannabis because of what's called the *entourage effect*: all cannabis compounds and terpenes work better when they're present together. Think about a symphony orchestra in relation to a single violinist. The single violin can sound good on its own, but the power of dozens of musicians working together creates a more majestic, emotional quality for the musical performance. This is what happens with the entourage effect. The cannabinoids and terpenes play off of each other and so tend to work better when ingested together. Many cannabis products are designed to leverage the entourage effect, because it's so powerful in creating the desired results.

MYRCENE

A terpene commonly found in mangos, lemongrass, hops (as used in beer) and thyme, on its own myrcene smells earthy, fruity and a bit reminiscent of cloves. Myrcene has strong antibacterial and antifungal properties and is one of the most common cannabis-derived terpenes. It is believed to promote calming and sedative "couch-lock" type effects (deep relaxation that keeps you on the couch). On average, myrcene represents about 20 percent of all the terpenes present in most cannabis strains today, which is why it's considered the most dominant terpene. Myrcene is found in strong cannabis strains like OG Kush, Grandaddy Purple, Blue Dream, and Cherry Pie. (Don't let those names throw you; we'll talk more about cannabis strains and their names later in this chapter.)

LINALOOL

Linalool is a terpene found in many plants, such as lavender and birch trees. In fact, it's so common in plants that most people end up consuming about two grams of it through their food every year.

Linalool has a floral aroma similar to lavender and is known to produce calming effects and relaxation. Overall, linalool is considered a rarer terpene in cannabis, because few strains contain very high amounts of it. Some cannabis strains known for linalool are Do-Si-Dos, Kosher Kush, and Zkittlez. Because of its antibacterial properties, linalool was once used as an antibiotic, and it has been used in traditional medicine practices for its sedative and anti-epileptic properties. Linalool may be less common than others, but it's an incredibly powerful terpene.

PINENE

If you have ever walked in a forest, you have definitely smelled pinene, the most abundant terpene found in the natural world. It has an aroma very similar to, you guessed it, the smell of pine trees. Along with pine needles, pinene is also found in aromatic herbs like mint, rosemary, and basil. It's useful for managing pain, inflammation, and anxiety. Pinene is also a bronchodilator, which means it opens the airways in your lungs. Pinene is an incredibly abundant terpene in cannabis plants. Thus, there are many cannabis strains that contain pinene, like Blue Dream, SFV OG, Cannatonic, and God's Gift.

BETA-CARYOPHYLLENE

Beta-caryophyllene is a major ingredient in rosemary, cloves, and hops. Its distinctive flavor is what gives black pepper its taste. It's a common and abundant terpene in cannabis. The scientific community has discovered that this compound activates endocannabinoid system (ECS) receptors, a significant medical discovery. Interestingly, beta-caryophyllene is the terpene that is detected by drug-sniffing dogs, since it's so ubiquitously present in cannabis. Beta-caryophyllene is reported to have anti-inflammatory, pain-relieving, and anti-brain-aging properties. Cannabis strains rich in it are believed to have high medicinal value because of this. Cannabis strains with high amounts of beta-caryophyllene include Bubba Kush, Sour Diesel, Chemdawg, Candyland, Deathstar, and Gelato #41.

An incredibly popular terpene found in lemon rinds, orange rinds, and juniper, limonene is often most evident because of its citrus notes. It's known for mood enhancement, stress relief, and antifungal and antibacterial properties. Some cannabis strains that contain limonene are White Fire OG, Lemon Tree, MAC, and Wedding Cake.

Cannabis Strains

Just as the tomato plants in your garden come in different varieties (Beefsteak, Early Girl, Roma), and dogs come in adorable breeds from Chihuahua to Saint Bernard, cannabis plants are classified into varieties called *strains*. Cannabis strains generally fall into three different categories: indica, sativa, and hybrid.

The strain classification is incredibly important when it comes to selecting the cannabis for you. However, it's really the source plant's cannabinoid profile that dictates the effects, and that can be affected by factors like climate, soil, and genetics. So be aware that your mileage may vary; a strain generally known for certain properties might not always deliver. Also know that in medical cannabis circles, different types may be referred to as "varieties" or "chemovars," since "strains" has a different scientific meaning.

Indica

Indica strains are characterized by the plant's dark-colored buds; short, dense structure; and short, wide, fan-shaped leaves. These plants have a deep relaxing effect, create a strong body buzz, and are often suggested for nighttime use. Users with high tolerances to cannabis often prefer indica strains. If you are a new user, it is important to know indica strains are commonly used as nighttime strains: think of indica as meaning "In da couch," a simple way to remember these strains are the heavy hitters that can leave you pleasantly reclining for a while. On the recreational side, these strains are for feeling super-stoned. On the medical side of things, if you are in pain or need help sleeping, you want to choose indica strains. In modern cannabis, most indica varieties have been bred to have almost no CBD content, in order to maximize the amount of THC that can be produced.

COMMON INDICA STRAINS:

- Bubba Kush
- Skywalker OG
- OG Kush
- Northern Lights
- Ice Cream Cake
- Purple Punch
- Grandaddy Purple
- Mendo Breath
- Platinum Kush
- LA Confidential

Sativa

Sativa plants are characterized by their tall, lanky structures and skinny, narrow leaves. Sativa strains are great for energy, focus, and creativity. People with anxiety may want to avoid sativa strains, because they are uplifting and can sometimes make anxiety worse. Sativas are typically sold for daytime use and are suited for physical activity, because they don't have the strong body high associated with indica strains. They can give almost the opposite of the deep relaxation "couch lock" effect commonly seen in many indica strains.

COMMON SATIVA STRAINS:

- Sour Diesel
- Green Crack
- Durban Poison
- Tangie
- Strawberry Cough
- Blue Dream
- Trainwreck
- Jack Herer
- Gorilla Glue #4
- NY Diesel

Hybrid

Hybrid strains are just that, hybrids of multiple strains. It does not necessarily mean that the strain is the result of breeding a sativa with an indica, although that is somewhat common. A hybrid strain can be the result of breeding indica and sativa strains together or maybe breeding two indicas or two sativas or two other hybrids in order to carry desirable traits.

Let's say you have a strain that's very beautiful in appearance, smell, and flavor, but it's a low-yielding plant. It would make sense to breed that strain with another strain that has a significant yield. The process sounds simple, but it can sometimes take years of selective breeding to end up with a plant that carries the traits that you want. Generally, the effects that hybrid strains produce are more balanced in nature. For example, you might have a sativa-dominant hybrid that's more functional and less racy and energetic than a pure sativa, so it could be used at night or more easily consumed by those who may be sensitive or suffer from anxiety. Hybrid strains can be both relaxing and energizing, depending on their specific genetics.

COMMON HYBRID STRAINS:

- Runtz
- Cherry Pie
- Biscotti
- Gushers
- Cookies and Cream
- Lava Cake
- SFV OG
- Sundae Driver
- Mimosa

THE STRAIN NAME GAME

Newcomers to cannabis often wonder about the names of cannabis strains and may be overwhelmed by the seemingly random and confusing way that cannabis has been named historically. The naming of strains has been an ever-evolving and controversial subject in the world of cannabis. Unlike some other plants varieties you might be familiar with (Big Boy tomatoes, Norfolk Island Pine Christmas trees), it's virtually impossible to identify a cannabis strain just by looking at it. Some do have distinct looks, but in general the naming of strains is based on many other aspects that are hidden from view.

Some strains are "landrace strains," named for where they were originally grown, such as Afghan Kush, which can be traced to the border of Afghanistan and Pakistan. Other strains are named after the plants that they were bred from; the name might be a literal hybrid of the strains used to create it. On the other hand, strains like Gelato or Cookies N Cream are named for their sensory experience. Maybe they do taste or smell reminiscent of ice cream or a sweet dessert! The gist of it all is, don't get too caught up in the sometimes playful, sometimes irreverent naming of the strains. Just be open-minded, ask questions, and do your research to find the products that fit your needs. One tip: follow your nose. It's been said that if something smells good to you, that may be a sign it's compatible with your body chemistry.

How We Use Cannabis

So now you understand that cannabis is a plant and that so much knowledge surrounding it is based on science, centuries of use and experimentation, and a ton of keen interest, passion, and dedication. But the real magic happens when our bodies interact with the compounds after consumption. There's a multitude of ways to consume cannabis, from smoking and vaping it to eating it or rubbing it on your skin. With legalization and the commercialization of cannabis, there are more ways now than ever, from beverages to transdermals (which allow cannabinoids to enter the bloodstream through the skin). Smoking, ingesting tinctures, and using topicals are seemingly the oldest and most common methods of consumption. But in recent years, there's been a shift toward new, nonsmokable consumption methods.

Women specifically have been driving cannabis into a wellness category, pushing topical and edible forms to become more common categories of consumption. Now that cannabis is legalized for medical or recreational use in over half of the United States, commercialization is driving innovation; thus, there are more consumption methods than ever before. There's even my company's namesake and family product, the Kush Queen bath bomb, for a bath infused with cannabis, as well as beverages of all types (cannabis wines, seltzers, and beers) for those looking for nonsmokable options. Let's take a closer look at the possibilities.

Inhaling

The most common way people consume cannabis is inhalation. We can inhale cannabis that's been vaporized (vaping) or combusted (smoking). Vapor is created by heating the cannabis flower or oil without combusting it. Combustion is what happens when we light the flower on fire. You can use a glass pipe or bong, or even roll a joint or a blunt with a tobacco wrap for combustion. Today, thanks to modern technology, much of the new use of cannabis is through vape pens or vape cartridges. These products hold cannabis oil or extract in a cartridge or a pod, then use a battery-powered heating element to rapidly heat up the cannabis and create a vapor ready to be inhaled.

Some consumers love the rituals of vaping or smoking. The grinding of the cannabis, the rolling of the joint, and the deep inhalation are all a part of their cannabis experience. However, some users are not interested in smoking because it's not a fit with their lifestyle. Plus, the reality is, cannabis is a very delicate plant with many volatile, sensitive compounds. And the best way to appreciate all of that is definitely not lighting it on fire, no matter how satisfying the results may be.

IS VAPING SAFE?

Most of the research around vaping is currently related to tobacco use and not cannabis. While a recent study found that vape cartridges may leak heavy metals, in states where cannabis use is legal, vape cartridges face strict testing for heavy metals, pesticides, microbials, and potency.

Edibles and Drinks

Americans have loved cannabis edibles since the 1960s (we love you, Alice B. Toklas), and many of today's users favor this nonsmokable way to consume cannabis. Legalization of cannabis has brought beverages of all types infused with cannabis, with wines, sodas, seltzers, and even beers are available in some places. In recent years edible cannabis consumption has greatly increased due to reports of vape-related lung illness and concerns about lung health during the COVID-19 pandemic. The variety of options for enjoying edible cannabis is nearly endless, with a myriad of products available: gummies, hard candies, chocolates, savory treats.

But there is a downside to edibles: you've got to digest them, and that process can be quite slow. On average, the effects of a cannabis edible or beverage can take about an hour to hit you. For some users, this isn't a good match. For others, getting the dose right can be a little more challenging, because with edible consumption, your liver converts some cannabinoids into more potent forms. So, it is incredibly important to understand that with edibles, you need to start low (the initial dose) and go slow (do NOT take more). You may not feel anything for an hour to an hour and a half; your body has to digest the cannabis, and that takes time. If you had a particularly heavy meal, that can slow the process down even further. Cannabis edibles and beverages produce significantly stronger highs than smokable or vaping methods. They are preferred by people who use cannabis for sleep because of the duration and the potential to be extremely sedative. Make sure you understand: once you take cannabis orally, you are locked in for a good four- to eight-hour experience.

Oils

Cannabis oils or concentrates are a more modern innovation, brought to us by technology. In the old days, cannabis oil was hash, which was extracted from the plant with ice water and then pressed to create the dark brown hash from long ago. Now, with modern techniques, equipment, and chemistry, we have many advanced methods to separate the good stuff (cannabinoids and terpenes) from the rest of the plant, creating amazingly potent and flavorful experiences.

Distillate, true to its name, has been distilled, or heated under vacuum and condensed in order to separate the compounds. The result is a purified oil that is comprised only of cannabinoids. The drawback is that all of the terpenes are removed, so others need to be added back to the oil before consumption for flavor and effect. Distillate is commonly the main ingredient in vape cartridges.

Solventless extraction processes take the old-school water-hash method and add micron bags and heated plates, physically squeezing and separating the oil from the hash. This is generally a top-shelf product that can have extremely powerful flavors and potent effects.

Solvent-based extraction products such as BHO (butane hash oil) can take the form of wax, shatter, sauce, diamonds, or sugar (named according to the form and appearance of the end product).

Whatever the extraction method, we're left with pure cannabinoids and terpenes. Some users prefer to vape these extracts; others prefer to eat them. All topicals, edibles, tinctures, and beverages are possible because of cannabis oil extraction.

Topicals

Cannabis topicals are one of the oldest ways people have used cannabis. Salves, body butters, lotions, body oils, lubricants, and serums can all be infused with cannabinoids. We call any type of cannabis-infused product that's applied to the skin a topical. A cannabis topical provides localized relief and is often chosen because of its nonpsychoactive properties. Due to the size of a cannabis molecule, cannabinoids placed on the skin do not get you high (even if the topical contains THC). But they can give you localized relief from pains, rashes, skin conditions, soreness, and inflammation, because our skin has many receptors that work with the endocannabinoid system (ECS). This makes cannabis topicals a popular category with women and with newcomers to the plant.

Tinctures

Cannabis tinctures are known as one of the healthiest and most approachable ways to consume cannabis. They are also one of the oldest ways people consumed cannabis as a medicine, because they don't require inhalation or combustion. Tinctures date back to the 1800s, when they were used to treat a variety of medical conditions. A cannabis tincture is a preparation of cannabis oil suspended in alcohol or a carrier oil. Nowadays, almost every tincture you will encounter is suspended in oil, although some still use alcohol.

We use a tincture sublingually, dropping it under the tongue and ingesting it. Some consumers enjoy mixing the tinctures into beverages or food, which will create a slower effect, since it sends the cannabis through your digestive system. A tincture placed under the tongue may have a quicker onset. But it's also possible the tincture won't be well absorbed and will be ingested more like an edible, with a 30- to 120-minute wait before the effects are felt.

Capsules

Cannabis capsules are a more modern innovation, available thanks to legalization. You can now get cannabis encapsulated in pill form! These are convenient for promoting sleep and for people looking for discreet, nonsmoking options. For those using cannabis for strictly medical purposes, they're a great tool for ingesting a specific dose. Some cannabis capsules have immediate release effects, and others are delayed or controlled-release. Capsules can be made using many different forms of cannabis, like oils, powders, isolates, and distillates.

As with edibles, capsules will be digested and end up passing through your liver and being converted into other molecules. This will increase the potency of the product, so please mind your dose; just as with edibles, start low and go slow. Some capsules may only contain CBD and no THC, so it's very important to understand that capsules are not one-size-fits-all. Make sure to pay attention to the details on the packaging.

Transdermals

Transdermal products are a result of the modernization of cannabis. While cannabis topicals have been around for hundreds, if not thousands, of years, transdermal technology in cannabis has only been around for the last few years. Ultimately, cannabinoids are not water-soluble, and their particle size is so large they cannot penetrate the dermis of the skin. Transdermals and transdermal technology use permeation-enhancing ingredients to allow cannabinoids to be absorbed through your skin and into the bloodstream.

This allows, for example, cannabinoids that are mood-affecting to penetrate the skin and get you high, unlike with traditional oil-based topicals. Transdermal products can be in the form of lotions, lubricants, patches, or creams and come in a wide variety of cannabinoid ratios.

GUIDELINES FOR USING CANNABIS SAFELY AND RESPONSIBLY

Cannabis has been used for thousands of years, but due to its murky legality and history, many have safety concerns. The reality is that no one has ever died from using cannabis, and some of its components in synthetic form are now FDA-approved drugs. According to medical cannabis advocacy group Americans for Safe Access, the Drug Abuse Warning Network Annual Report's statistical compilation of all drug deaths in the United States has never reported any deaths from the use of cannabis. In 1988, DEA chief administrative law judge Francis Young said, "In strict medical terms, marijuana is far safer than many foods we commonly consume . . . Marijuana in its natural form is one of the safest therapeutically active substances known to man."

Of course, everything and anything can have a downside or be abused. Cannabis does have a small list of risks you should be mindful of as you begin to integrate it into your lifestyle. Some effects that you want to be prepared for include coughing or wheezing (if cannabis is inhaled), euphoria, dry mouth, reddened eyes, increased appetite, blurred vision, dizziness, headache, delayed motor reactions, sedation, and anxiety. These are short-term and could last on average for two to four hours, unless you have indulged in edibles whose effects can and will last longer. The presence of these effects can vary from person to person, and these can also be affected or heightened by the setting where you consume or what delivery or consumption method you are using.

The longer you use cannabis and the more you build a tolerance, the more likely these side effects are to subside or the less likely you are to feel them. Most of the negative effects of cannabis have to do with chronic use by inhalation. Since you are a newcomer to cannabis, you should know (like with everything) it's best to use in moderation. As a long-time user, I recommend following these rules for safe and responsible use of cannabis:

1. Never drive or operate heavy machinery while high or while consuming cannabis.

2. Never mix edible or ingestible cannabis with alcohol. (I have done it, and I promise you don't want to do it.)

3. Start low and go slow. Give edibles at least two hours before you re-dose.

4. Always store your cannabis in a safe place, away from children and pets.

5. While cannabis has a very limited list of known pharmaceutical drug interactions, you should always consult your doctor before using it if you take prescription drugs.

6. Do not use synthetic cannabis of any kind.

CHAPTER 2

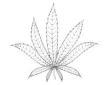

The Benefits of Cannabis

NOW THAT YOU UNDERSTAND ITS HISTORY, molecules, consumption methods, and risks, it's time to dive into the best part of the cannabis plant: the benefits! Most likely your curiosity about cannabis stems from hearing about all the wonderful things the plant can do for people. While the FDA has only approved cannabinoids for a few specific diseases and disorders, there have been countless studies over the past several decades that have shown a variety of significant and impressive benefits. As soon as I integrated cannabinoids into my own wellness routine, my health flourished. I have since developed my relationship with cannabis, and I'm excited to share with you everything that I have learned. Women especially have so much to gain from this powerhouse of a plant.

What We Think about When We Think about Cannabis

One of the things that led me to be successful in cannabis and understand it deeply was that I didn't grow up inside a procannabis bubble. As a kid in South Louisiana with family in both law enforcement and medicine, I knew all the anticannabis arguments very well. In junior high school I was a DARE kid; in South Louisiana we all had to participate in Drug Abuse Resistance Education, which taught only fear and danger around this plant (and still teaches anticannabis education to children). At age 14, when I saw someone use cannabis for the first time, I cried and immediately told my mom.

My parents were not hippies or farmers, but they were secretly using cannabis for most of my childhood. Then, when I was 18 years old, I finally experienced for myself what the plant has to offer. As I got older, I was able to build my own firsthand experiences, touching, using, growing, and extracting the plant. These experiences led me to understand the full extent of the stigma that cannabis users are working against. That's when my views truly softened, and I understood the complexities of the cannabis plant. Cannabis sits at a strange intersection as a social justice issue, a medicine and wellness tool, and a means of connection (to oneself and others).

The longer I use cannabis, the more I understand how our views of it actually change our experience. In DARE, we were taught that all drug use has inevitable, repeatable outcomes, but now we understand this is not the case. "Pharmacological determinism," an idea brought to the mainstream and criticized by journalist Hamilton Morris, is the flawed and disproved idea that a certain drug will always do a certain thing. We can see the failed war on cannabis and other drugs has caused irreparable harm that the plant itself could not be capable of. History has shown this medicine to be used by people of all races, ages, and socioeconomic statuses; yet its criminalization has been a tool of oppression against Black and brown people. Even in 2021, Black Americans are over three and a half times more likely than white Americans to be arrested for cannabis use.

All of this historical stigma casts a shadow over our cannabis use today and can make the experience feel scarier than it is. As you dive into this journey I hope you suspend your fear, which can and will affect your experience with this plant. If you're ever able to see cannabis grow from a seed to a beautiful plant and watch it flower, you'll know that the pain, fear, and issues surrounding the plant were caused by humans. The nature of cannabis is gentle, giving, and healing. When it is approached with understanding, knowledge, and respect, you can experience all the benefits. So take a deep breath, and let go of any stigma you may be carrying.

The Medical Applications of Cannabis

The medical community has had an interesting relationship with cannabis. Harvard Medical School's Kevin Hill explains, "We're conditioned as physicians to believe that cannabis is bad for you, but there is data that it can be useful in certain cases." Now with three FDA-approved drugs containing synthetic cannabinoids, we have begun to see a shift happen. More and more physicians and others in the medical community are coming to embrace cannabis. Some of the best and most promising work on the medical side was spearheaded by parents of children like Charlotte Figi, one of the most prominent figures who inspired the CBD movement. She tragically passed in 2020 from COVID, but her story truly transformed the medical community's perspective on cannabis.

Sanjay Gupta, chief medical correspondent at CNN, publicly changed his stance on medical use of cannabis in part because of his firsthand experiences with Charlotte. She was a child with Dravet syndrome who was having over 300 seizures a week until her mother researched and pursued cannabis medicine for her. The strain bred for her was named Charlotte's Web, and as other children began to also have success with it, her story captivated the world. Another

American hero, Sophie Ryan, has been living with a brain tumor since she was eight months old. She has paired traditional Western cancer treatments and brain surgery with medical cannabis. She's now almost 10 years old, and her story has had an extremely profound influence on physicians and the medical community. It's led many to evolve their thinking around not just cannabis as medicine but the science behind it.

Thanks to the impact of these people and others, we're seeing physicians and the medical community open up to cannabis as a medicine for epilepsy, cancer, even for treating the opioid epidemic and the mental health crisis. We're finally seeing thousands of articles perpetuating the war on drugs and lies behind cannabis removed from the National Library of Medicine. As the research restrictions are lifted, we will continue to see medical research expand and the medical community further embrace this medicine.

What Cannabis Can—and Cannot—Do for You

Over the last 10 years, we have seen cannabis barrel into commercialism, for better or for worse. Now cannabinoids are in everything from pillows (yes, there's a CBD-infused pillow on the market) to lubricants. For years, I have been a vocal opponent of putting cannabinoids into just anything and everything. At the end of the day, cannabinoids should enhance a product, and their inclusion must make sense. For example, a sexual lubricant with an anti-inflammatory molecule that can increase blood flow to increase sensation does makes sense. On the other hand a CBD-infused pillow, which means the cannabinoids can't be absorbed, just doesn't make sense. It concerns me that these kinds of gimmicks can cause people to believe that CBD or cannabis is a joke or snake oil, perpetuating the stigma and keeping the medical community skeptical. So I'll continue to protest. In the meantime, as a cannabis consumer it's important you arm yourself with knowledge to discern what products are actually utilizing these molecules effectively.

Cannabis can't fix everything and anything under the sun. But what it can do, especially when paired with Western medicine, is what's truly important. During my own cannabis journey, I used cannabinoids to help wean myself off of long-term pharmaceutical use. The cannabis did not get me off of the prescriptions on their own, of course, but it did aid in alleviating my symptoms as my body withdrew from eight long years of daily medication. My 21-year-old cousin is a quadriplegic with cerebral palsy. Since integrating cannabis with his medications and therapy, he's had a significant reduction in spasticity and in the negative side effects of some of his medications on his digestive tract. When my aunt was dying of cancer, she used cannabis to ease her pain and treat the symptoms of chemotherapy. The molecules in cannabis aren't a cure-all, but they pair incredibly well with modern Western medicine. If you manage your expectations and understanding, you will set yourself up for better success using this special plant for medical purposes.

Why Women Use Cannabis

Women have always used cannabis in history, and their use in modern times is rising. For example, NBC News reports that Gen Z women are becoming the fastest-growing segment of cannabis users. That resonates, at least symbolically, because only the female cannabis plant produces flowers. So, in other words, all of the cannabis we consume is female. Women use cannabis for countless reasons, but many are driven to cannabis to help manage monthly menstrual cycles and the pressures women face in their personal lives. Of course, all genders use cannabis for a myriad of purposes. But it's women who've driven CBD and cannabis into the wellness conversation. We will dive much deeper into this in part 2 of this book, but here are some of the many reasons why women use cannabis.

IS THAT FACT OR FICTION?

Due to the war on drugs and the antidrug movement it created, misinformation around cannabis is staggering. When you see some of the articles once available in the National Institutes of Health and the National Library of Medicine, you can understand why cannabis was once such a divisive issue in the medical community. Scientific journal articles that have been proven to be funded and pushed by anticannabis groups have been widely discredited and removed from databases. There is simply overwhelming evidence that cannabis use is not as harmful as we were taught for nearly a century.

It is so important to be able to discern the propaganda, divisiveness, and misinformation around cannabis. Understanding that the loudest voices often sit on the opposite ends of the spectrum is important. Here are some prominent myths and truths you should be aware of.

Cannabis use has not killed anyone, ever.
Fact. There isn't one recorded death directly from cannabis to date.

Cannabis is not addictive.
Fiction. It is important to know cannabis can be addictive. Is it as dangerous as fentanyl, as once claimed? Absolutely not. But have people developed cannabis dependency? Absolutely. It's essential, as with anything, to use cannabis in moderation.

Dose matters.
Fact. When it comes to some of the claims perpetuated by antidrug groups, the size of the dose is often completely left out of the conversation. The size of the dose of

cannabis is incredibly important in relation to both positive and negative effects. Microdosing cannabis (taking small amounts), especially as a beginner, can remove the risks of taking too strong a dose.

CBD cures all.
Fiction. CBD is a molecule that holds much promise and power, but it is not a cure-all. It can't cure cancer and doesn't reverse the effects of unhealthy things you put in your body. Anyone claiming benefits to pouring CBD on everything is surely spreading misinformation.

Cannabis is less harmful than alcohol and tobacco.
Fact. The numbers don't lie with this one. Alcohol and tobacco have caused far more societal harm and health issues for users than cannabis use.

Chronic and Acute Pain

The pain pathway of the endocannabinoid system (ECS) is lined with receptors that interact with cannabinoids—the cannabis molecules fit into these sensors like keys in a lock. People have been using cannabinoids for pain management for thousands of years. THC's power as an analgesic and CBD's impressive anti-inflammatory ability can have a truly transformative effect on managing pain, especially when combined with the entourage effect in mind.

Stress

Stress relief is one of the most common reasons women come to cannabis. From mothers to white-collar professionals, women love cannabis as an approachable means of managing stress. The COVID pandemic only added to this phenomenon; in one poll reported by *Bizwomen*, 8 in 10 cannabis consumers have found the drug to be helpful for managing pandemic stress. According to statistics, women are just overall more stressed out than men, so it makes sense that women have taken to the healing and gentle nature of cannabis to manage it.

PMS

Women have been using cannabis for PMS and menstrual pain since ancient times. From tinctures to topicals to edibles, women appreciate the relief brought by the power of cannabis as their monthly cycle arrives. Muscle aches, cramping, nausea . . . our cycles arrive with symptoms that cannabinoids can successfully treat. So it's only natural that women use cannabis as a plant-based alternative for treating PMS and other related issues.

Endometriosis

Over 176 million women worldwide reportedly suffer from endometriosis. The endometriosis community has long used cannabis for symptom relief, and there's great hope it can also treat the underlying condition. Mounting evidence is showing that cannabis can stop the spread of detrimental endometrial tissue growth.

Fibromyalgia

Just like endometriosis, fibromyalgia is a disorder women face for which cannabis shows a massive amount of promise. According to a Healthline report, in a 2011 study, approximately 43 percent of participants who used cannabis for fibromyalgia reported strong pain relief and 43 percent reported mild pain relief. Fibromyalgia greatly affects women's ability to sleep, which is also why so many turn to cannabis.

Skin Conditions

Cannabinoids hold an anti-inflammatory power that make them an incredible tool for skin care. From body oils to CBD face serums to bath bombs and body lotions, cannabis skin products have become a hot category in the beauty space. Celebrities like Kim Kardashian use CBD and cannabis skin care for psoriasis and eczema. Remember, the skin is your body's biggest organ, and it's full of receptors that interact with the endocannabinoid system, which makes cannabis and skincare a match made in heaven.

Sex

Cannabis is a known aphrodisiac and great for pain. So women often find themselves reaching for cannabis when it comes to sexual health. From relieving vaginal and postchildbirth pain to just increasing blood flow to the vulva to increase sensation (yes, that's why it works so well), cannabis offers powerful support for a satisfying sex life. Some women love a puff before doing the deed, to relax deeper into their bodies; others choose a cannabis-infused lubricant to add to their sex routine. Many women experiment with CBD lubricants postpartum for recovery and pain management.

Mental Health

A recent study found depression was less prevalent among cannabis users; this may be one clue to why women love using cannabis for mental health. Over 246 million people worldwide suffer from depression, and many find cannabis pairs well with pharmaceuticals. Research suggests women use cannabis for mental health and in conjunction with pharmaceuticals (largely to reduce side effects) in large numbers.

WHERE MORE RESEARCH IS NEEDED

It's rather surprising to most cannabis newcomers that until recently, medical research involving the plant was so severely restricted that it was effectively banned. Since 1968, only one US facility has been granted the necessary license from the National Institute on Drug Abuse (NIDA), which was a long-running hindrance to all US cannabis research. Now that this restriction has been lifted, there's an abundance of medical research being done. The biggest space where we need medical research on cannabis involves minor cannabinoids. There is so much unlocked potential with these compounds, and due to their more targeted effects, understanding them could yield countless therapeutics for specific diseases.

For example, there are a few incredibly promising studies with the cannabinoid THCV for weight loss, diabetes, and obesity. With obesity such a significant health issue in America, more research in this area could have a huge impact on public health. The same goes for cannabinoids that seem to improve sleep, a cornerstone of good health and wellness. If research confirms what anecdotal evidence and citizen science show, there could be hundreds of millions of people who could benefit. Or consider the opioid epidemic, which has affected millions of people. Pain management medication offers very few therapeutics without a significant risk of addiction; cannabinoids might serve that need. There are also the areas of cancer and autism; cannabinoids have shown significant promise in treating both diseases (in fact, there are currently millions using cannabinoids to treat them). With more medical research, we could see life-saving breakthroughs that could save and improve so many lives.

Wellness

There's a significant movement of women using cannabis for overall wellness, a trend driven by and for women. The wellness conversation now considers cannabis as a valid option, along with meditation, breath work, and yoga, for preventive wellness. From a daily intake of CBD to the ritual use of cannabinoids in self-care routines, significant anecdotal evidence suggests that cannabinoid use has an important impact on overall wellness. Cannabis use and wellness both have the same outcome in mind, after all: feeling our best. So it's no surprise women are championing cannabis for wellness not just when disease or disorder is present but as a preventive health measure.

Sleep

Over 70 million Americans struggle every day with sleep and sleep-related disorders. With changes in hormones, high stress, perimenopause, and menopause, women make up a significant portion of the millions whose sleep issues bring them to cannabis. THC and CBD have been shown to be of great benefit in helping women fall and stay asleep, with fewer side effects than pharmaceutical sleep aids. Sleep sections are common in cannabis dispensaries, offering products specific to helping consumers get a great night's rest. While the science is a mixed bag, there is an undeniable reality that cannabis helps many enjoy restful sleep. And a substantial number of people engage with the plant specifically for that reason.

CHAPTER 3

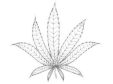

The First-Timer's Guide to Buying Cannabis

BACK IN 2007, WHEN I WORKED AT A MEDICAL cannabis dispensary, times were simpler and so was our stock. We offered flowers, homemade edibles, and hash. Today when you walk into a dispensary, you'll see hundreds of products. It's actually pretty overwhelming, especially if you're new to cannabis. As a former budtender, I found that working at the dispensary was where I truly fell in love with cannabis and the people who use it. In this chapter, I will help you navigate the world of buying cannabis and all it entails.

First Things First: Is It Legal?

Welcome to the world of legal cannabis! Legalization is about much more than not being arrested for using cannabis; the term is actually about regulations around the growing, sales, manufacturing, distribution, and use of cannabis in your state. Currently, 19 US states have legalized recreational cannabis use (in order of legalization: Colorado, Washington, Alaska, Oregon, California, Maine, Massachusetts, Nevada, Michigan, Vermont, Illinois, New Jersey, Montana, South Dakota, Arizona, New York, Virginia, New Mexico, and Connecticut), as well as Washington, DC, and Guam. Some of these states, like New York and South Dakota, have only recently legalized adult-use consumption. So in New York there is no regulatory framework for the growing, buying, and selling of cannabis, but you can legally consume it while rules and regulations are being developed. These regulations often take years to create and execute.

Legal cannabis has become a burgeoning industry, providing consumers access to safe, lab-tested, and fully regulated cannabis products. Gone are the days when you had to feel scared or put yourself in danger to acquire cannabis. The industry has also become a significant job and tax revenue creator. Cannabis legalization is happening state by state, but there has been very little movement at a federal level. Thus, you can legally acquire and consume cannabis in one state, but you cannot travel with it across state lines. As a new cannabis consumer, you need to try to educate yourself on your state's regulations to the best of your ability and follow federal progress as well. Federal laws may not affect you as a consumer, but they affect the legal industry in a myriad of ways. These laws also keep an estimated 40,000 people convicted of nonviolent cannabis crimes in prison, for doing what people do in the legal cannabis market every day.

Let's dive deeper into what is actually legal, the process for accessing medical cannabis, and how to be an ethical cannabis consumer.

It's Actually Not Legal to . . .

Even though cannabis is legal for recreational or medical use in 37 states, that doesn't mean it's legal to do everything with it. Driving under the influence of cannabis is illegal, no matter where you are. And from a safety standpoint, it's important to never drive or operate heavy machinery when using cannabis.

You should never transport cannabis across state lines, even if you're traveling from one cannabis-legal state to another legal state. The biggest thing to know is that the laws are different in every state. For example, in California you can legally consume cannabis anywhere smoking is allowed, except for federal property. But in Washington there is absolutely no legal public consumption. One day when the federal laws change, we may have a unified set of rules. But until then it's up to you to do your own research.

These activities are illegal even in states that have legalized cannabis use:

- It's illegal to travel with cannabis across state lines.

- It's illegal to share cannabis with minors.

- It's illegal to drive while under the influence of cannabis.

- It's illegal to bring cannabis into a national park or onto any federal property.

- It's illegal to ship cannabis in the mail.

Your First Trip to the Dispensary

The cannabis dispensary has evolved quite a bit since the days when I was a budtender. There are now many more different types of products and experiences, not to mention the driving force of commercialization. It's no surprise that a dispensary visit may be intimidating to a first-timer. I would go with you if I could. But I can do the next best thing and talk you through it.

CAN I GET A MEDICAL CARD?

In my state of California, we have legalized recreational cannabis, but I still hold a medical use card. That's because in California you can get a lower tax rate and purchase larger amounts with a medical card. Ultimately, my cannabis consumption is for medical use, so I will always have a medical card.

When it comes to accessing medical cannabis, there's a general framework you can follow if it's legal your state:

Medical cannabis cards normally require a **qualifying condition**. So the first thing you want to do is find your state's list of qualifying conditions. These are typically listed on your state's health department website.

Next, you need to **find a doctor** qualified to issue medical cannabis cards. Some states may provide telemedicine access for this. The doctor will ask you some basic questions about your condition and do an evaluation. Some may inform you of the side effects of consuming cannabis. The doctor will decide to grant you the medical cannabis card if you're a good candidate. It could take a few days or a few weeks for the card to arrive in the mail, depending on your state.

You may need to **register your medical card** before you go to a dispensary. Most states, like New York and Connecticut, require patients to register with the state health department. In California, you don't need to register a card or join a database. Once the card is issued, you can visit a medical cannabis dispensary. In any case, remember to bring your card!

The first and most important thing to bring with you to a dispensary is your government-issued ID card, a driver's license or the equivalent. There's no way to get into any dispensary without it. The other big tip is to bring cash, or a debit card so you can draw cash from a nearby ATM. Despite all the progress, and some dispensaries looking like Apple stores, most still have no access to banking. Thus, 99 percent of them remain a cash-only experience.

A majority of dispensaries display their products in glass cases and will assign a budtender to guide you through your shopping process. Dispensaries typically carry cannabis flowers, prerolled joints, extracts, varied edibles, and topicals. Due to regulations, you most likely cannot touch or smell the cannabis flower. In fact, you should manage any and all expectations to sample or touch any products. The inventory is frequently held in back areas for security.

Medical and recreational dispensaries may differ in the types of products they carry. Most medical dispensaries have higher-dose products than what's allowed in recreational stores. Medical dispensaries may have more rare cannabinoids or less common extracts, like Rick Simpson oil (a full-spectrum extract with extreme potency, normally reserved for cancer patients and the terminally ill). Another big difference will be the price. Recreational dispensaries will almost always have the highest prices and taxes.

Most budtenders will start by asking you whether you came in for anything specific or have a current ailment you are trying to treat. (Remember that budtenders are not trained medical professionals. Be sure to confirm any medical advice with a doctor.) If you are interested in smokable cannabis, expect them to inquire about your preferred strain or the effect you are looking for. The best budtenders have sampled a vast majority of the products available and have a palpable knowledge of the plant. Unfortunately, some budtenders are not that experienced or knowledgeable. Worse, some may get kickbacks for selling you certain products. This is another reason to start low and go slow until you land on a product that meets your needs.

WHY LEGALIZATION MATTERS

Within the last 10 years we've seen a massive shift in not just the perceptions around cannabis use and decriminalization but also legalization. With legalization, not only does cannabis use become legal, but its growth and sale become regulated. This means that legislators and regulators put in place frameworks (rules, licenses, testing requirements, and the like) that keep consumers and young people safe and also contribute tax dollars to infrastructure.

While the legal industry may not interest you as a consumer, there are a few key points I believe every cannabis consumer should understand.

- Buying cannabis from a licensed producer is safer, because regulatory bodies require strict lab testing.

- Buying legal cannabis contributes tax dollars to education, infrastructure, and law enforcement.

- Statistics show that fewer young people get access to cannabis in places where it's regulated and taxed.

- In some places, cannabis tax dollars provide money to formerly incarcerated people who were impacted by the war on drugs. In other places, social equity programs put communities that were disproportionately affected by the war on drugs at the front of the line for licensing or charge them lower fees, so they can participate in legal cannabis.

- Buying legal cannabis can be more expensive than buying unregulated cannabis, but the higher price is because of the regulations and taxes.

The Ins and Outs of Purchasing Cannabis

After all these years, going to the dispensary is still my favorite part of being a cannabis user. It's like Disneyland, but for adults. Bring your sense of fun with you; your cannabis experience begins the moment you walk in the door.

The best part of the modern dispensary experience is that the days of not knowing what you are buying are long gone. The dispensary will be organized, and more important, the products you will be buying will be safe and lab-tested, and the potency of the product will be clearly labeled (though specific testing and labeling requirements vary by state).

A big shock to first timers isn't the products themselves but the way they're packaged. It's an unfortunate side effect of regulated cannabis; be prepared for bulky, high-maintenance packaging. Most regulators have mandated childproof or child-resistant packaging for safety. It's why we say the buying of cannabis is easy; it's the opening of the cannabis package that's hard.

Before heading to any dispensary, make sure to check the menu on their website or a third-party site that offers updated menus of local dispensaries. These stores often do high volumes of sales and have an ever-changing selection. Do not assume they will have a well-stocked inventory; always check before you leave home. This is also my pro tip for getting the best prices. Dispensaries are fully aware that cannabis is a luxury for most people. They are constantly running promotions, specials, and deals for customers to take advantage of. Never leave home without checking the online menu!

Let's take a closer look at what's inside those glass cases.

FLOWER

Cannabis flower is the OG (original gangster) of all cannabis products; it is the classic experience for a first-timer. You will likely see dozens of different types of indica, sativa, and hybrid flower. Each jar or bag of flower should be labeled with its strain name and potency. Dispensaries will offer the dried flower or prerolls (prerolled joints) by weight. So be prepared to understand whether you want a gram (1 gram), an eighth (3.5 grams), a quarter (7 grams), a half ounce (14 grams), or an ounce (28 grams). Remember, if you buy dry flower, you will need a pipe, bong, or rolling papers to smoke it. I recommend starting with a few grams each of different strains. This way you don't have an abundance of a strain that doesn't work for you or that you don't like. If you would like to experience flower without needing paraphernalia to consume it, opt for a prerolled joint. Dispensaries will have an abundant selection of prerolled cannabis for those pursuing lower-maintenance options.

You'll want to shop by strain, because that's what will likely produce the desired effect or get you the results you're looking for. Dispensaries will absolutely have the potency posted or available to you. But do not get tripped up on potency; the most important thing when buying any kind of cannabis flower (prerolled or not) is the freshness. You should ask your budtender for the harvest or packaging date. In all my years of experience, the best cannabis wasn't the highest potency, it was the freshest.

CONCENTRATE

In my experience, the concentrate section may be the most overwhelming for newcomers. It's certainly not the usual place to start, because enjoying most cannabis concentrates requires additional technology to heat them, like a vape pen or a dab rig. However, cannabis concentrates are definitely the purest, strongest expression of the plant. Although there is a lot of fear around dabbing and its high potency, just like with anything, you can definitely use a tiny amount and get a fantastic effect and flavor. (I suggest a small amount, the size of the tip of a nail or a ballpoint pen.) You will see the products here named by strain and potency, just as in the flower section of the dispensary. But unlike in the flower section, the extracts sit in tiny jars labeled with a ton of new words you most likely haven't heard before. Most of the concentrate names will refer to the consistency or the way the concentrate was processed. For example, "live resin" refers to a concentrate that was made with a fresh-frozen plant (a plant frozen immediately after harvesting). "Budder" refers to a concentrate that has a softer consistency, with a look and texture like butter. "Rosin" refers to a solventless extracted concentrate. While the media has vilified this type of consumption, concentrates are a very potent and tasty way to enjoy cannabis. Just as with edibles (coming up next), using them is all about education, approach, and dosing. So proceed with extreme caution or wait until you're further along the cannabis path.

EDIBLES

The edibles section is one of the fastest-growing areas of cannabis dispensaries. Check it out and you'll see gummies, chocolates, beverages, candies, powders, cookies, and more. Most recreational markets cap edible products at 100 mg total cannabinoid content and require the products to be dosed around 10 mg per serving for safety. Even then, that dose may be incredibly high for a newcomer. Remember to start low and go slow. If you are looking for edibles to help you sleep, keep an eye out for ratios and CBN products that are geared towards sleep. With commercialization, we've seen a massive increase in lower or microdosed edible products. These products are often perfect for those new to cannabis and can be dosed anywhere from 2 to 5 mg of THC per serving. Remember, the ingested cannabinoids will convert in your liver, which will increase their potency and length of effect. Edibles are the best choice for people experiencing severe pain and sleep issues. Just remember to try them at home, where you're safe, and with a sober friend staying with you the first time.

OILS

Pure cannabis oils will be readily available at a dispensary. Some will be for body use and will be found in the topical section. Other oils are edible and in tincture form. Some oils will be pure cannabis oil that's in a carrier oil like MCT oil. These will be perfect for adding to your food or smoothies. Some people just don't love the hempy taste of cannabis, so there's a wide variety of oils and tinctures that contain flavorings or aromatic essential oils. These products are perfect for sleep and good choices for people who aren't interested in consuming the sugar or calories found in edibles. Many oils and tinctures will be classified by their cannabinoid ratios or minor cannabinoid content. These are highly recommended for people looking to integrate cannabis into their daily routines.

IT'S ALL IN THE RATIO

"Ratio" refers to a blend of cannabinoids that helps you reach your desired effect. Most ratioed cannabis products are blends of CBD and THC, but some can be blends of other minor cannabinoids. Ratios range from greater than 20:1 all the way to 1:10. A general rule of thumb is that anything with a dominant CBD to THC ratio of 10:1 should not create a high effect.

TOPICALS

Your skin is your body's biggest organ, so never underestimate the importance of cannabis topicals. The dispensary will have balms, salves, lotions, creams, lubricants, body oils, and (I hope) my own original cannabis product, the cannabis-infused bath bomb. These products are all going to be infused with cannabis oil, and frequently they're paired with essential oils for targeted effects (the entourage effect again). Not all dispensaries have large selections of topicals, as they're one of the smaller segments of the market. But do not undervalue the potential of these products to help with your menstrual cycle, injury recovery, skin health, and overall wellness. Remember to check the ingredients if you have any skin allergies.

CAPSULES

Capsules are an excellent choice for consumers looking for smoke-free or more medicinal options, like improving your sleep or help recovering from an injury. The capsules come in many forms and may have a few different looks. From a golden distillate gel cap to pressed tablets, they're a good reminder of how far we've come from buying dry cannabis flower in zip-top bags. There will be capsules with blends of both CBD and THC; some may offer ratio options like 10:1 or 20:1 (10 or 20 mg of CBD to 1 mg of THC), which are perfect ratios for new users to try. The blend of CBD and THC can mitigate side effects like paranoia. There may also be unique cannabinoids, like THCA (tetrahydrocannabinolic acid) capsules, which can deliver some benefits without a high at all. Dispensaries often have minipacks of five capsules or larger 30-day supplies once you have found your favorite capsules.

TRANSDERMALS

The world of transdermals is fairly new, so manage your expectations when it comes to finding a vast selection. When shopping for these, be sure to ask your budtender specifically for transdermal products. The scientific definition of a transdermal is an application of a drug through the dermis of the skin. So these products will be used to deliver cannabinoids into the body. Traditional topicals, in contrast, do not cross the skin and enter the bloodstream, so they cannot get you high. There will be patches, lubricants, lotions, shower gels, and maybe, if you're lucky, cosmetics. When you are buying a transdermal, the available potencies may appear to be lower. For example, nontransdermal lubricants are often dosed with a 100 mg potency, but a transdermal lubricant may only be 30 mg or 50 mg. Why? The technology of transdermal products increases the bioavailability of their compounds. You absorb more of the cannabis, so a transdermal can have a stronger effect than a topical with a higher potency. Another reality of transdermals is that they may be more expensive than regular oil-infused topicals. If you can afford them, it is my experience that transdermals work substantially better than traditional topicals, especially pain relief and sexual lubricant products. Some transdermal products may be labeled with terms like nano, nanoparticle, or nanotechnology.

WHAT IT MEANS TO BE AN ETHICAL CANNABIS CONSUMER

As a woman who's worked in the cannabis industry for the last 15 years, I encourage you to be an ethical cannabis consumer. Why? Well, the legal cannabis industry is predominantly run by white men and large corporations; your purchasing choices can support independent business owners and diverse cannabis providers. I also hope you consider engaging in activism around cannabis (see the Resources section, page 139, for suggestions). Policy at the federal level remains unclear and over 40,000 people (disproportionately people of color) remain incarcerated for cannabis-related convictions.

What does being an ethical cannabis consumer look like? Once you are deeper into your cannabis journey, consider researching the brands you support. While the industry has seen an overall increase in minority workers, we have a very big diversity problem at the stakeholder, C-suite, and executive levels. Your ethical cannabis decisions will help make the cannabis industry just as diverse as the people who use cannabis. Ask these questions, and favor brands that can answer "Yes."

- Is this brand operated by women, LGBTQ+, or BIPOC owners?

- Does the company support reparations and record expungement, or participate in community engagement for incarcerated cannabis users?

- Does the company encourage ethical employment practices?

- Does the company engage in transparency around the workforce?

So . . . What Do You Want? A First-Timer's Frequently Asked Questions, Answered

Q I've never gotten high before, and I'm curious but also a bit nervous. Where should I start? What do you think I should avoid?

A The first thing you must decide when trying cannabis is what delivery method you prefer. Do you want to smoke it? Eat it? Rub it on your skin? Do you have pain, or are you treating a specific disorder? If you're looking to just give it the old college try, buy a preroll and try a joint for the first time. It will have the shortest duration of high, and it's the most low-maintenance way to get started. Take a few deep breaths and try to suspend your nerves before you light her up. From my 15+ years of dispensary experience, I think it's best for beginners to avoid edibles and concentrates, unless you cannot (for health or personal reasons) smoke or inhale cannabis. Edibles and concentrates are some of the most potent options in the dispensary, and it's important that you understand that getting too high too soon can ruin all the fun of exploring cannabis.

Q What's the number one question to ask a budtender when buying flower for the first time?

A Remember that freshness is the most important thing when buying flower. Do not get stuck with last year's weed (yes, it happens sometimes). Ask your budtender for the harvest date, and you will have the best cannabis experience. Most budtenders may guide you by THC content, but this is a rookie move. The number one question, and the only question I ask a budtender when buying flower or prerolled cannabis flower products, is "What is the harvest date?"

Q What if I only have a limited budget?

A Cannabis is still a luxury for some. If you have a fixed or strict budget, make sure to inform your budtender. That way they won't show you products that are out of your price range, which will speed up the process. Taxes also play a major role in the cost of cannabis. Ask the budtender whether the tax is included in the price to avoid choosing options outside of your price range. You can check a dispensary's online menu for sales and promotions.

Q Can I bring someone with me when I go to shop at the dispensary?

A In most recreational dispensaries, you simply need to be 21 with a valid ID to enter. In some medical dispensaries, you will need to have a medical card to enter. Don't be shy about calling ahead of time to figure out whether you can bring a friend.

Q If I don't like a product, can I return it?

A Dispensaries and brands have varying return policies. In some states, the laws block returns altogether. In states that allow returns, dispensaries will have many different policies. Familiarize yourself with the dispensary's return policies before you buy. In my experience, if I could not return a product, frequently I'd contact the brand directly. Often they'd find a way to replace it or provide some sort of reimbursement for the bad experience.

Q Do you need to tip the budtender at a dispensary?

A It's standard at dispensaries to see a tip jar on the counter. Tipping is of course encouraged, but tipping budtenders is not yet an established norm. As a former budtender, I always tip my budtender when they provide me great service, guidance, or extra attention in helping me find what I need. Consider how much you are spending on the cannabis when you are considering the amount to tip, as well.

Buying Legal Products Outside of a Dispensary

In 2017, the cannabis industry experienced what will forever be known as the mainstreaming of hemp CBD. I witnessed firsthand the shift in public perception of hemp-derived CBD and the legal changes that would follow. In 2018, the US government legalized hemp CBD under the Farm Bill. The 2018 Farm Bill determined that plants with under 0.3 percent THC would be classified as hemp, and any cannabis plant with over 0.3 percent THC would be classified as nonhemp or cannabis. Hemp cultivation and production were expanded nationwide, ushering in a major hemp boom. Now there are thousands of hemp CBD companies, and CBD can be found in airports, gas stations, hemp dispensaries, pharmacies, cosmetics stores, and grocery stores. In some places you can get a manicure and pedicure with hemp CBD; in others you can enjoy a latte with a dose of CBD.

Even though hemp CBD is legal, it is currently unregulated. This means that as a consumer you need to arm yourself with knowledge and only choose the best products. Due to the unregulated nature of CBD, consumers can buy products that are mislabeled, underdosed, or even contain no CBD at all. The FDA has been discussing regulation of CBD products but has yet to make any rulings. Until CBD is fully regulated, you must choose reputable companies that make consistent products and prioritize transparency.

Buyer beware of gimmicky products like CBD pillows and burgers; the market has become a Wild West of companies putting CBD in virtually everything. The reality is that CBD as an active ingredient does make sense in many products, but you need to think critically about the why of the product. For example, with a pair of CBD-infused yoga pants, how would the CBD be absorbed into your skin? It wouldn't. So it's important to ask yourself whether a product makes sense or not.

Never ever select a CBD product that doesn't make lab tests or COAs available. A COA, or certificate of analysis, is a lab test of the product's CBD content. It's the only way to know a product is accurately dosed and safe for consumption. Here are some guidelines to follow:

- Look for lab-tested products with certificates of analysis or lab tests available.

- Choose products with potency clearly indicated on the front of the product label.

- Be aware that many companies frequently mislabel hemp seed oil products as CBD.

- Look for products that detail the specific type of CBD (e.g., isolate, broad spectrum, full spectrum).

- Look for products with a supplement panel (the panel of information found on vitamin and supplement packages).

- Look for products that include the manufacturer and the date of manufacture on the label.

In part 2, we'll explore CBD products and their uses more deeply.

CHAPTER 4

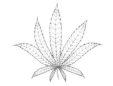

The First-Timer's Guide to Getting High

SO NOW THAT YOU'VE GOT THE GOODS, WE'LL dive deeper into the specific applications of cannabis—starting with the art and act of getting high. If I had told my 18-year-old self that I would be writing this chapter one day, she would have never believed me! When it comes to getting high, experience is sort of everything. So one could say all the times I got high were just advanced training for sharing my knowledge with you. This chapter will prepare you for everything else that comes along with getting high for the first time.

What It Feels Like to Be High

Dry mouth, red eyes, and the munchies . . . you've probably heard the clichés. It's time to talk about what it really feels like to be high. Broadly speaking, getting high is simply changing your consciousness and heightening your senses. But all cannabis highs are not the same, despite the way movies and TV have portrayed them. Some highs are deeply relaxing; some help you feel deeper in your body. Sometimes you find laughter in ways you didn't know you could laugh. And other times, yes, you get the munchies. The one thing that getting high isn't, is the same experience every single time.

The biggest thing to understand about using cannabis to get high is that no two highs will ever be the same. Sure, you will frequently experience some of the same side effects, like feeling thirsty, changes in perception, and appetite stimulation. But you have so much control over your high and the type of high you experience. For example, as I write this chapter I am feeling a light sativa buzz, bursting with energy and creativity from a few puffs of a joint. Later tonight, when it's time for a movie, I'll find that laughter-filled, lazy, super-stoned state, thanks to an indica edible. Just as there are endless strains of cannabis, there are endless types of experiences.

All of the information in part 1 of this book can guide you to the high you are looking for. The strain and terpenes will have a large influence on the type of high you experience, as will your delivery method and dose. There are many other factors that can affect your high, like whether you had a big meal or indulged in alcohol before consuming. Your current state of being and current mood may affect your high and experience, too. Another major factor may be whom you are with and where you are. Cannabis isn't just a plant, it's an effect and an experience, which can be affected by many variables.

Even besides all that, cannabis affects each and every person differently. You could enjoy cannabis with a friend and not feel the same things from the same strain or product. The endocannabinoid system is completely unique to each of our bodies, like our fingerprints. Thus, cannabis does not work exactly the same way every single time with every single person. Your hormones, your lifestyle choices, and your DNA can and will affect the way your body interacts with cannabinoids.

Naturally, there are some basic misconceptions and myths about cannabis. For example, some people believe cannabis makes you hallucinate. Surely, at a massive dose (over 100 mg of THC) hallucination is possible, but it's unlikely if you start low and go slow. Many cannabis users, especially those new to cannabis, are scared off by the paranoia they experience. If you have too much or use too high of a dose, you can experience paranoia. But I often coach people that this effect could be due to the way we think about cannabis. Our fear of it can create paranoia in the experience. With the right dose, delivery method, and setting the intention of a positive experience, you can help the outcome of your cannabis high.

Bottom line: all highs are not the same. So let's unpack and explore some of the most common types you can experience with cannabis.

"I don't feel hazy, I just feel good."

One could say this may be the best type of high, even though that's an incredibly subjective judgment. You feel euphoric, optimistic, hopeful, and happy. Your senses are heightened; your energy buzzes with all that is good. This experience can provide you with mental clarity and a feeling of peace. The world may look brighter and almost movie-like. You may feel like a social butterfly or more connected to nature. This type of high will leave you feeling carefree, like you left your worries behind. Some parts of your body may feel heavy, but your mind feels liberated. The greatest highs of this type will leave you feeling like the best, most supercharged version of yourself.

"I'm sorry, but I can't stop laughing."

There is nothing like a session that leaves you laughing so hard you cry. With cannabis, it's very possible to experience laughter or joy unlike anything you have ever felt before. I have genuinely woken up the next day with sore abs from the incessant and uncontrollable laughter of a high like this. You may find yourself finding something that's usually unfunny to be completely hilarious. You may find a movie or joke funnier or more laugh-inducing than ever. Or that you've never had the giggles like this before. It's a feeling where you just can't stop laughing at something, which only gets harder when you try to make it stop.

"I'm having trouble getting up off the couch."

Welcome to the world of couch-lock. This when your high feels deep in your body and makes you feel glued to the couch. This is much deeper than ordinary relaxation, and it's perfect when you want to shut out the world or literally do nothing. Most frequently, this high is achieved with edibles or ingestible cannabis, but some smokable strains can accomplish it, too. While some people may hear "couch lock" and feel like it's negative, the phrase simply refers to the deep, beyond relaxation level of the body high. It's perfect for a lazy weekend or rainy Saturday. Make sure to have snacks, because this type of high will absolutely come with a case of the munchies, and you won't want to go anywhere for food.

"I'm feeling oddly productive"

Some newcomers to cannabis may be shocked that you can unlock a productive and active high, but it's one of my favorites. With the right strain selection (sativa or sativa-leaning hybrids) and delivery method (vapes and prerolls), you can unlock a high that is energetic and active. Some cannabis users love to unlock this high before organizing or cleaning. Others will pair it with exercise. After all, it's been discovered that "runner's high" is due to your endocannabinoid system, caused by endogenous (naturally occurring in the body) cannabinoids.

"I'm feeling creative."

For centuries, artists, musicians, and creative people have been known to use cannabis to tap into their creativity. You may find yourself wanting to write a poem, paint a picture, or even color an adult coloring book. There's something magical about unlocking your creative high. Some refer to this type of high as a "head high," meaning you feel it more in your mind than in your body. Cannabis is known to heighten your perception, increase your senses, and improve focus on a task. For some people, this combination yields a flow state, or a heightened state of creativity. Ideas flow more easily, colors look more vivid, and you may feel more connected and free in your creative thinking.

"I'm feeling enlightened."

One of my favorite cannabis experiences is when it helps me see a different perspective or brings a sense of enlightenment. This type of high can bring an "A-HA!" or light bulb moment. Your state of relaxation and changing your consciousness can bring a new perspective on a situation. Sometimes you'll have an unexpected epiphany. This type of high isn't commonly discussed, because so many people perpetuate the idea that consuming cannabis will just leave you stoned and unable to think. But mounting evidence shows cannabis can increase blood flow to the brain, including to the frontal cortex where our higher-level thinking occurs. This can cause us to experience new perspectives, better problem-solving skills, and improved thinking on a subject. Sometimes when I'm faced with a problem, I decide to smoke on it. This type of high can also be achieved if you consume cannabis and meditate.

THE CANNABINOID THAT DOESN'T GIVE YOU THE MUNCHIES

Back when I was a budtender, customers sometimes asked for specific strains known anecdotally to have the opposite effect of the munchies, suppressing the appetite instead of stimulating it. Since those days, not only has our good friend science located a skinny-girl cannabinoid, but a few medical studies have found that it shows great promise. Meet THCV (tetrahydrocannabivarin), the appetite-suppressing cannabinoid.

THCV is a molecule predominantly found in sativa-dominant strains. As its name suggests, THCV is similar to THC in molecular structure, and it has the potential to be euphoric like THC at high doses. But at lower doses, THCV provides a variety of altogether different effects, which users describe as euphoric, uplifting, energetic, motivating/focus-inducing, and appetite-suppressing. Those who have used THCV have reported stress relief and a reduction in panic attacks.

There are different types of THCV: delta-8-THCV and delta-9-THCV. Research points specifically to delta-9-THCV for these exciting benefits. So when shopping for THCV products, it's important to read and understand the lab tests. You should look for:

The type of THCV in the product. Medical research specifically mentions the use of, effects, and benefits of delta-9-THCV.

The amount of THCV present. You want to make sure you are getting the molecule as advertised, not a watered-down product or a product with high amounts of THCV. Look at the total milligrams of THCV used compared to the total milligrams of the product.

Ummm . . . Is This Working? A First-Timer's Frequently Asked Questions, Answered

Q **This is my first time using cannabis; I don't want to get too high but I DO want to get high. What should I take?**

A Great question! Here's what I recommend if you can buy a prerolled joint, look for a FRESH one (harvest date and manufacture/packaging date will be listed on the packaging, which you can always ask to see before purchasing). And I recommend an indica-leaning hybrid strain like Runtz, Gelato #41, or maybe Wedding Cake. If you can't find a good preroll, you can get the same experience with some flower and a small glass pipe or a bubbler.

Start by taking just one single deep inhalation. You do not want to keep the smoke in your mouth; that isn't going to get you where you want to go! Breathe the smoke slowly and deeply into your lungs, and exhale. Some people say that you need to hold the smoke in for a long time, but that isn't necessary and can make you cough more. Now, just wait a few minutes. Maybe get up, move around a little, go grab a glass of water. You will feel a slight shift in your conscious awareness and perception. After about 10 minutes, any effects that will come should already be there. How do you feel? Is it strong enough? Then you're good for at least an hour or two. If not, repeat the same steps. For your first time, just go slowly and take it one toke at a time, and you'll never get too far out.

Q I want to try edibles for the first time, but I've heard horror stories about people getting way too messed up. What should I do to prevent this?

A Yes, it's known as the classic green-out, bug-out, or *the dark place*. And it's not something to take lightly. So here's what you do: use a technique called microdosing. Normally, edibles will come in servings of 10 mg. If that doesn't sound like much, the truth is it can be *quite potent*. Let's say you have a chocolate bar with 10 pieces that contain 10 mg each, or a bag of gummies that are dosed the same. For your first time, I recommend cutting that single dose into quarters, so you end up taking only 2.5 mg. Use a knife to cut the gummy or chocolate into four pieces that are equal in size, and just eat **one**. I know, it's probably delicious. But trust me, in an hour or so, you will start to feel the effects. At this microdose level, you will almost certainly not get too high.

Q I've been drinking a bit; should I smoke or eat an edible right now? Sounds like it would be really fun.

A Absolutely not! This is how you get into the classic "cross-fade" condition, also known as "the spins." It's a sure-fire way to end up on the floor, throwing up, sweaty and pale, or in any number of various bad states. Combining alcohol and cannabis should be considered strictly prohibited for a new user.

If you're farther along on your journey, and you have built a tolerance to cannabis, the safest way to try this is to get high first, then get a little beer buzz going. But if you're fairly intoxicated from alcohol of any kind, and you hit a joint or a bong—or even touch an edible—no matter your tolerance, the likelihood that you will feel sick and probably ruin your evening is significant. Mixing psychoactive substances is tricky and can lead to suppressing of effects, as well as your body rejecting what's going on entirely, causing you to vomit or possibly black out. Be careful out there!

Q I'm going on a hike, and I want it to be a high hike. What do you recommend as far as what to consume and when?

A Since you are a new user and your tolerance is low, I suggest bringing a vape pen along (you don't want to bring any flames into the wilderness, as it's a fire hazard). This will allow you to take a few hits when you're getting started, and you can discreetly puff as needed throughout the experience, effectively titrating your dose and controlling the strength of the high. Often the physical exertion of a hike can make the high wear off more quickly, so be aware of that. Also, since it's likely earlier in the day and you will be doing a lot of physical activity, this is a good time to try out a sativa strain if you have been nervous about trying one before. Get out, enjoy nature, and explore your surroundings, your senses, and your inner self!

Q I just smoked a joint, and I'm about to meet some friends for dinner, but I don't want to smell like weed. Any tips?

A Yes, there are a few things you can do. First, you need to wash your hands very thoroughly. Your hands likely smell quite a bit more than anything else, since cannabis smoke does not tend to stick to your clothes like tobacco smoke can. Then we focus on the mouth. Use some mouthwash or a breath strip, or just brush your teeth. If your hands are clean, your breath is clean, and you've let yourself air out a bit, you should be good to go. Now, if you still have some fresh, high-quality cannabis in your purse or pocket, that will definitely turn some heads. So if you're going for discretion, leave your stash at home or locked in your car trunk, and you're on your way to stealth mode.

MUSIC AND MOVIES:
A STONED GIRL'S BEST FRIEND

When we are high, our senses are heightened and our consciousness is elevated, so enjoying music and movies with cannabis is a perfect pairing. Film, TV, and music aren't just great to enjoy with cannabis; they have also driven forward normalization and progress.

Here's my go-to playlist of songs to get high to and my favorites to watch when I'm imbibing. All of the songs are about cannabis in different ways. Some of the TV shows and films are classic stoner comedies, and others have iconic pro-cannabis moments. Check these out and create lists of your own!

Playlist

- "Slow Burn," Kacey Musgraves
- "Watermelon Sugar," Harry Styles
- "Yes I'm Changing," Tame Impala
- "Sativa," Jhené Aiko
- "Girl Blunt," Leikeli47
- "Mary Jane Holland," Lady Gaga
- "High by the Beach," Lana Del Rey
- "Mary Jane," Rick James
- "James Joint," Rihanna

Watchlist

- *Broad City* (TV show)
- *Weed the People* (documentary)
- *Smiley Face* (film)
- *Clueless* (film)
- *High Maintenance* (TV show)
- *Rolling Papers* (documentary)
- *Dude, Where's My Car?* (film)
- *Sex and the City* (TV show)
- *Empire Records* (film)

What to Do If You Have a Bad High

There's nothing like a good high for nurturing your relationship with the cannabis plant. The reality is, however, that bad highs or experiences do happen. I've been high thousands of times, and I've only had a handful (literally only two times that I can recall) of bad experiences, all brought on by overconsumption or the wrong dose. We've discussed some of the side effects of getting high previously, but it's important we dive deeper into the negatives so you can understand what to do if it ever happens to you.

If you have a bad high, you are most likely too high. Less commonly, you may find a particular strain that doesn't agree with you. Or maybe you indulged in alcohol or caffeine with your cannabis (I don't recommend that). But what does it *feel* like? Most bad highs will carry paranoia and anxiety. There is something incredibly specific to the type of paranoia cannabis can produce, because your senses and consciousness are heightened. Additionally, cannabis is a vasodilator, so it can increase blood flow. In my experience, this can sometimes feel like anxiety, and it can also make you sweat a lot. If you're having a bad high, you could also experience confusion.

It's so important to understand the rarity of these experiences and that they will always subside. One of the most essential things you can do is to not panic, because panicking can exacerbate the situation. Infrequent "green-outs" (taking too much cannabis) or bad highs are just a part of the territory. Nonetheless, if it happens to you (or a friend), these are my tips for handling things.

Just Breathe

Take seven long, slow breaths in and out. Focus only on your breathing. Inhale slowly, and exhale slowly. Our breathing is one of the most powerful tools to rely on when we need to focus the mind. As you breathe, remind yourself: cannabis has never killed anyone. By resetting with seven long, slow, deep breaths, you can reconnect and reset your experience. By breathing and simply focusing on inhaling and exhaling, you can absolutely breathe your way through a bad high.

Eat Food and Drink Water

Hydration, hydration, hydration! This is a major tactic for managing a bad high or green-out. Stick with water or juice, and please avoid alcohol or caffeine (both can increase the effects of THC). Hydrating will help with your dry mouth and allow you to focus on something outside of being super high. Eating a snack like fruits, nuts, and cheese is another tool for grounding a bad high.

Sniff Black Pepper

Remember when we talked about terpenes in chapter 1? This is a terpene-based way to chill your high. You will want to activate the smell, so crush or smash a few fresh peppercorns. Then move your nose close and take a careful sniff. Inhaling the actual pepper can be unpleasant, so be cautious, or try chewing a few peppercorns instead. This method is excellent for people experiencing extreme paranoia. Just a fair warning, you may need to sneeze postsniff!

Make Lemon Juice

Limonene is another well-known terpene that can diminish a high or ease a bad high. It's known to modulate THC's effects on the body and brain. Luckily, lemons are packed with limonene. If you find yourself too high, squeeze some juice from a fresh lemon, or zest a bit of the peel, then add a little bit of sugar. Then drink it or consume it to combat your bad high.

KEEP IN MIND

We've reached the end of part 1, having explored the experience of getting high for the first time. You now know the types of highs, the negatives to look out for, and what to do if you feel things have gone too far. When you feel nervous about all this, remember that cannabis has never killed anyone and is an incredibly gentle plant. You are armed with knowledge that will recreate the outcome you desire. Here are the most important principles to follow.

Relax. Remember that your experience with cannabis is heavily influenced by how you feel about it. The way you feel about cannabis can affect your high, so stay positive whether you're alone or with friends.

Focus on the setting. Your setting will always play a significant role in getting high. Using music or creating a supportive space to get a better high is key. Have your playlist, comfiest clothes, snacks, and all you may need nearby and ready.

Be prepared. Just because we're getting high on cannabis doesn't mean we're lazy or unprepared. You know yourself, and you know what will make you feel comfortable and safe, so take appropriate measures. You also want to prep your cannabis as needed before you dive in.

Know your limits. Remember to start low and go slow. You can always take more, but you can't take less once you have consumed it. You can't go backward, so consume carefully.

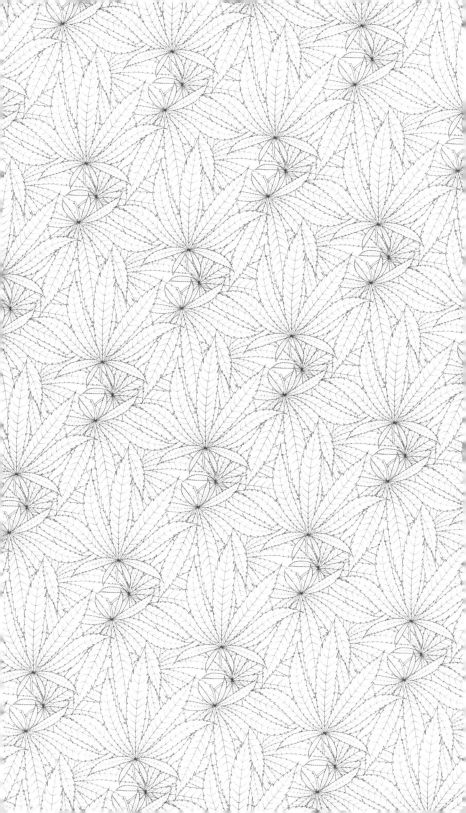

PART 2

PRACTICAL APPLICATIONS OF CANNABIS

ANNABIS IS AN INCREDIBLE plant, but without us, it's just a plant. Cannabis becomes magic when we learn to apply it in our life and feel our endocannabinoid system come alive. In this section, I'll share my knowledge with you as we walk through the practical benefits that cannabis can bring. I'll give you the whys and hows, and I'll leave you with some pro tips. What you do with this knowledge will be up to you.

CHAPTER 5

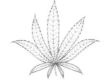

Mental Health

THE LAST 15 YEARS OF MY LIFE HAVE BEEN dedicated to developing cannabis products for mental health, and it's the number one reason I use cannabis every single day. I have used this plant to wean myself off eight years of pharmaceuticals for my own bipolar disorder. This is where I feel so much of cannabis culture and information is missing and frequently overlooked. Yes, access is opening, but there is a gaping hole in *how* and *why* cannabis has a role to play in managing mental health challenges. Specific cannabinoids can be used for treating anxiety, stress, depression, ADHD, PTSD, insomnia, bipolar disorder, opiate dependence, grief, and even, in some cases, schizophrenia. When treating mental health issues with cannabis, it is important to work with a mental health professional who can support your journey.

It's also crucial, if you are on pharmaceuticals, to speak with your doctor about consuming and using cannabis.

Since California's Proposition 215, which passed in 1996 and gave us medical cannabis in California, there has been a much wider acceptance of cannabis as therapy for mental health issues. Now that we better understand the role the endocannabinoid system plays in mood, stress, appetite, and cognitive thinking, it makes total sense that cannabis can be used as a therapeutic for mental health. That being said, some cannabis compounds should be approached cautiously for mental health applications, specifically THC and other psychoactive molecules that can further induce anxiety or create further risk for people predisposed to psychosis. As we explore this topic, we'll dive into the best delivery methods and approaches for cannabis use in relation to different mental disorders.

First, some general principles. Whatever you choose to take, when you begin your journey with cannabis for mental health, please remember to stay consistent: stick with something for at least 30 days. Mind your dose (most medical research shows less is more when it comes to cannabis and mental health), and remember to listen to your body. When approaching cannabis for mental health, we also need to be mindful of our caffeine and alcohol consumption and understand possible interactions with any pharmaceutical drugs we're taking.

Your body is incredibly sensitive when mixing these molecules with cannabis. As you move through your journey with cannabis, make sure to check in with yourself. Remember that our environment is ever-changing, and our approach to cannabis should be, too.

What to Use

Now that you've gotten a high-level overview of cannabis use for mental health, it's time to dive into specifics. In this section we will get detailed in considering which cannabinoids can be used for best results. When using cannabis for mental health, it's important to pay attention to the cannabinoids themselves, as some are better fits than others, especially when it comes to mental illness.

For Anxiety

Anxiety is one of the most common reasons people come to cannabis for mental health. Those with anxiety should always take oral CBD (capsules, tinctures, or edibles) daily, something that has been known to improve anxiety in all doses. Additionally, THC in micro and small doses has been known to improve anxiety as well. But understand that THC in high doses can trigger anxiety, so those with anxiety should always mind their doses of THC in order to avoid making anxiety worse.

For an Overactive Mind

The best known cannabinoids for ADHD are THCV (tetrahydrocannabivarin) and CBG (cannabigerol). Indica strains can help those experiencing an overactive mind. Those with ADHD will definitely want to mind the strain and terpene profiles. I recommend a 1:1 THC:CBD ratio to start, in edible or tincture form. Hybrid strains and sativas can help with focus. Indica strains can help with hyperactivity.

For Stress

Daily CBD use can greatly aid in lowering stress levels in the body, specifically full-spectrum CBD. Another great tool for stress relief is microdosing. Look for products with only 1 to 2 mg of THC in them. Vaping is also a great solution for those using cannabis for stress. Approach high-THC strains for stress with caution; they may make you feel more stressed.

For Depression

Depression is best approached with high CBD and low THC. Medical research shows this can assist with depression. Over the long term, high THC can make depression worse, so look for high-CBD strains like Charlotte's Web or ACDC. For depression, a ratio of 20:1 CBD:THC is a great choice. I recommend at least 30 mg of CBD per day to start. Remember that the dose that works will vary based upon your diagnosis, weight, height, diet, and lifestyle.

Look also for the cannabinoid CBG (a.k.a. cannabigerol, or the "bliss molecule"), the chemical precursor to CBD, which has the most street cred when it comes to cannabis and depression. Citizen science says it holds great promise for treating depression.

For Grief

With grief and cannabis, it's important to be guided by your needs at the moment. Maybe it's getting a good night's sleep, stimulating appetite, or taking the edge off after holding it together all day. Being mindful about how you feel and what you need in the moment is key for choosing the best product.

Pro Tips

Plant medicine alternatives like cannabis can be great tools for your mental health. But at the end of the day, they are only as good as your knowledge of how to use them. I know these practices will help guide you in healthy, helpful choices.

✓ Do load up on CBD.

If you are using cannabis or cannabinoids for mental health, it's incredibly important to have CBD every single day. The consistent daily use of CBD has been known to alleviate stress, anxiety, and a host of mental health issues. The best results will come from consistent use, even if you feel no effects—that doesn't mean it's not working. Checking in with your body and learning to listen to it will guide your cannabis journey. If you're under added stress, adjust your dose. If you are feeling lethargic, dial it back. Cannabis is not one-size-fits-all, and monitoring its effects will help you develop a greater sense of mind-body connection. Even now, after 15+ years of using cannabis for mental health, I am always learning and experimenting.

✓ Do speak to your doctor if you are on pharmaceutical medication.

If you are taking any medications, DO speak with your doctor about using cannabis, even if you are scared to! You never want to put your health at risk. Cannabis can cause interactions, and it's important to be honest with your physician if you're consuming cannabis.

✓ Do look for minor cannabinoids.

As the science evolves, minor cannabinoids are turning out to hold even more promise for supporting mental health than THC. Give the minors like CBN (cannabinol), CBG (cannabigerol), and CBDA (cannabidiolic acid) a try, if you can find them. Some of these molecules may become the next mental health superstars.

✗ Don't play with high doses of THC.

Most of the science says that very high doses of THC, or high doses of psychoactive molecules in general, don't work best for mental health. High doses of cannabis can cause more mental health negatives than positives. Using high doses of a cannabis product can induce further anxiety and even psychosis. The science shows that for mental health, low THC is more effective (we don't eliminate it completely because of the entourage effect). I would be wary of THC doses higher than 10 mg per serving. Most recreational markets do not allow the sale of edibles with higher doses than that.

✓ Do explore microdosing.

Most of the science around mental health shows that cannabinoid microdoses are the best bet for treating many mental health disorders. Microdoses (1 to 2.5 mg) will be less psychoactive. And you can always go up in dose if you're not feeling results, but you cannot lower the dose once you take it.

✗ Don't consume THC if you're in active trauma or experiencing high anxiety.

If you are in an anxious or active trauma state where you are actively experiencing high emotion from an event, you should not consume any THC. It can absolutely exacerbate your feelings and make the situation worse.

✓ Do mind your setting.

The space and setting where you consume is always important when using cannabis (or any drugs with psychoactive properties). I recommend only consuming cannabis in a safe space or environment. A safe space can be in your own home, the home of a trusted friend, or even a peaceful outdoor setting that's comfortable and private. Being with people who make you feel safe, removing distractions by turning off your phone, and keeping to a place free of interruptions or strangers can help improve your high.

Frequently Asked Questions, Answered

Q **I've been using cannabis to treat my anxiety for a few months. It's working, but I'm still experiencing symptoms. Should I change my routine?**

A Always be evolving your routine. Our environment plays a major role in our mental health. So do the seasons. I'm always changing my own routine and tweaking my dose. For example, during the fall-to-winter transition, I up my dose of CBD by at least 25 to 50 mg. This helps me adapt to the seasonal changes, like the clocks changing due to daylight savings time (does *anyone* like this?).

Q **I have been dealing with a lot of stress/anxiety, and I find myself unable to sleep lately. I sometimes toss and turn for hours. What can I do to help this?**

A Even people without a history of sleep disorders or insomnia, when triggered by anxiety or traumatic events, can find themselves struggling to get quality sleep. Here's what I recommend well before your desired bedtime, shut off all screens (TV included). Play some calming, ambient music, and make sure your bedroom is the right temperature and as comfortable as it can be. At least an hour before bed, take a healthy dose of CBD (try 15 mg), and if you have it available to you, take about 5 to 10 mg of CBN in addition to your CBD dose. Once you're in bed, try to focus on relaxing each part of your body, one at a time, starting with your feet and moving your attention slowly upward. Focusing on your breath (the flow in and out and how it fills your lungs and deflates them) can also help you drift off to sleep. If you are able to get to sleep but cannot stay there for more than a few hours, consider trying a transdermal patch before bed to extend your sleep.

Q I need a mood boost during the day. I don't know whether I am depressed, but I feel like my brain could use a kickstart to get some more happy juices flowing. What would be the best product to take?

A I would start by experimenting with products containing high levels of CBG. Many users report an elevated, blissful-type effect when consuming this molecule specifically, and I agree completely with those reported effects. I like to describe CBG as almost making you feel *lighter*. You get that little boost, pep in your step, whatever you want to call it. It really works to elevate your mood and can really help brighten your day when you're feeling down and dark. I don't recommend taking CBG too late at night, as it can have a bit of a stimulating quality for some and may interfere with getting to sleep when you need to.

Q I have a specific mental illness and racial trauma. My doctor refuses to talk to me about it. How can I find information or support from people that are experiencing similar issues?

A When it comes to Western medicine, we often encounter a one-size-fits-all approach and that one size tends to be centered on the white male experience. In my experience, the best information on applying cannabis to a specific side effect or disorder is often found peer-to-peer. It may be as simple as connecting with a Facebook group through search terms like "Black women who use cannabis for anxiety" or "corporate women who use cannabis." For me, finding people who were using cannabis for bipolar disorder was the defining moment in my care. The group I found provided me with community support and made me feel it was safe to ask questions my doctor simply couldn't answer. There is something so special about the community element of cannabis, even if it's digital. Feeling seen, feeling heard, and being supported by people who understand your struggles is priceless. It's also an incredible source of information when it comes to strains, delivery methods, and approaching mental health with cannabis.

Takeaways

- If you are actively on pharmaceuticals for mental health, consult your doctor about interactions before using cannabis. Always talk to your doctor, therapist, or psychiatrist about your cannabis use.

- Find a support group to connect with others currently using cannabis for your disorder. Whether the group is online or in person, some of the best information on dose and delivery method specific to disorders is shared peer-to-peer.

- Always be checking in with yourself, journaling, and evolving your routine. Our bodies are always changing because of our environment. This way you can find patterns and monitor your intake to get the best results.

CHAPTER 6

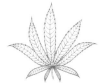

Aches and Pains

AS I SAT DOWN TO WRITE THIS CHAPTER, I thought about my own experiences using cannabis for pain. It occurred to me that I don't often take over-the-counter pain relievers like ibuprofen or Tylenol, or even experience a lot of pain generally, but I am a daily cannabis user. A few nights ago, I felt a nerve in my foot ache, and I soothed it with a nanoparticle-based cannabis lotion that took the pain away nearly instantly. I thought about my weekly ritual where I soak in a cannabis-infused bath bomb, which leaves me feeling like I went and got a full-body massage. I could go on and on about how I reach for this plant whenever I have aches and pains. According to a Pain News Network report on a recent Harvard study, after six months of daily treatment with cannabis, patients experienced significant improvements in their pain, sleep, mood, anxiety, and quality of life. On average, their use of opioid pain medication decreased by 13 percent and 23 percent after 3 and 6 months of treatment, respectively.

The CDC reports that over 50 million Americans suffer from chronic pain every day. Cannabis is an increasingly popular alternative to OTC medications and opioids for pain management. From chronic pain to pain from nerve damage and inflammation, there's an ever-evolving world of cannabis use for pain management of all types. Since ancient times, women have used cannabis for menstrual pain, and now we have a wide variety of cannabis products for pain of all types. So let's dive into the cannabis strains, delivery methods, and doses used for pain relief.

The pain pathway of our spine is lined with endocannabinoid receptors that help modulate pain inside our bodies. The opioid epidemic has surely pushed cannabis for pain into the spotlight, as it does not carry the same risk of addiction, overdose, and harmful side effects that opioids do. Moreover, cannabis is also a better alternative for the body than NSAID medications like ibuprofen, as they are known to cause liver damage when used consistently over time.

A 2015 review of research on the use of cannabis and cannabinoids for various chronic pain reported that several trials had positive results. The researchers suggest that cannabinoids can be effective in treating neuropathy or nerve pain. Another research paper from 2016 found that cannabis use for chronic pain led to a 64 percent reduction in opioid use, improved quality of life, and caused fewer medication side effects. Generally, it also led to participants using fewer medications.

Many doctors remain skeptical about cannabis for pain, but there are two synthetic cannabinoids that the medical community has begun to prescribe off-label for the treatment of pain. My hunch is that in the coming years the FDA will approve many more synthetic cannabinoids for pain management.

Pain is a very general term, so let's touch on some of the most promising scenarios in which cannabis can help you:

Neuropathic pain. A recent review of all medical science relating to cannabis for neuropathic pain (nerve pain) found THC to be an effective treatment.

Migraine. When it comes to migraines, cannabis is both preventive and abortive. One study found participants had far fewer migraine attacks if using inhaled or edible cannabis. A clinical trial found that "cannabinoids are just as suitable" to prevent migraine attacks "as other pharmaceutical treatments," in the words of a report in the *European Pharmaceutical Review*. It appears dose is a significant factor; most people need around 200 mg of a 1:1 ratio product.

Nausea related to pain. Extreme pain can cause nausea and vomiting, for which cannabis often provides great relief. Specifically, delta-8-THC is known to be the very best cannabinoid for fighting nausea. A study on pediatric cancer revealed that delta-8-THC was successful in preventing vomiting completely when the participants were undergoing chemotherapy.

Chronic pain. The THC in cannabis will help temporarily relieve pain by reducing the body's pain signaling and pain perception. Chronic pain stemming from physical and systemic inflammation, such as rheumatoid arthritis, may benefit from the anti-inflammatory effects of cannabis as well. CBD specifically may help.

What to Use

One of the most positive aspects of the commercialization of cannabis and the expansion of the industry is that the pain-relief section of most dispensaries is more evolved than ever. You can stick to the traditional route and find a number of smokable strains great for pain management. But now there is so much more available than just flowers. The dose, delivery method, and strain will all make a difference when it comes to cannabis for pain. There are salves and lotions, often paired with essential oils for pain relief. There are edibles for those experiencing more serious or severe chronic pain.

There are even cannabis-infused vaginal serums and lubricants for treating vaginal pain and endometriosis. Migraines, spasticity (muscle tightness), fibromyalgia, arthritis, and nerve pain are all frequently discussed and treated with cannabis.

When it comes to cannabis for pain, you may want to use a few different delivery methods, depending on your pain level. For example, when experiencing pain recently, I didn't just smoke cannabis, I combined it with topical and edible cannabis. You want to mind your tolerance, and always start low and go slow. But combining delivery methods can greatly aid in relief.

Topicals are a perfect tool for body pain, arthritis, and general aches and pains. Some may prefer salves or oil-based topicals. For more serious pain and deeper penetration, look for nanoparticle-based topicals; these are transdermal and are the most effective for pain management. Transdermals do often have a higher price tag than traditional cannabis salves. Oil-based topicals (not transdermal) cannot get you high; if you choose these types of products, consider higher doses if you have the budget.

Pain patches are a new cannabis-infused product you may see in dispensaries. These transdermal patches are great for injuries, menstrual pain, and the pain experienced by cancer patients. The patches can be placed on the skin, and this delivery method inherently allows an extended duration of effect.

Capsules and tinctures are two more of my most highly recommended tools for those experiencing chronic or more serious pain. Of course, dose and ratio of cannabinoids will matter.

For those in serious pain, smoking cannabis can help immensely. Here are my recommendations:

Best Strains for Pain

Heavy indicas and strains with caryophyllene (a great terpene for pain)

- Daikini Kush
- Pure Love
- Blue Zombie
- Flaming Cookies

- Skunk Ape
- Matsu
- North American Indica

- Fallen Angel
- Double Purple Doja

Pro Tips

When it comes to cannabis for pain, the biggest thing to understand here is the dose. As a newcomer to cannabis, it's important to mind your dose, because we don't want you to get too high and have a bad time. But the truth is with pain, you often need to explore cannabis in higher doses or ratios. People with conditions that cause pain often have extremely high tolerances to cannabinoids and require higher doses to feel the effect. This doesn't mean you shouldn't proceed with extreme caution. It just means you may end up with a higher dose than for other uses.

✓ Do choose high-THC products over high CBD-products.

For pain, THC just seems to work better than CBD. When it comes to THC, there's delta-9-tetrahydrocannabinol and delta-8-tetrahydrocannabinol. The THC most people know is delta-9-THC, but recently delta-8-THC has exploded because of its ability to be sold as a legal hemp product outside of the regulated cannabis markets. Both will work for pain; access to one or the other will likely depend on where you're located.

✓ Do start low and go slow.

You will build a tolerance to cannabis, like other pain modalities. So, starting as low as possible is key.

✓ Do explore and combine delivery systems.

For example, dose 5mg of edible cannabis after breakfast and dinner, and then use localized topicals on the area where the pain is present.

✓ Do explore transdermal topicals for pain.

These have increased potency, get absorbed more quickly, and work faster for relieving pain.

✓ Do explore products with other ingredients for pain.

For example, products with essential oils for pain, pain relieving herbs (e.g., turmeric, clove, willow bark, capsaicin), or cooling effects (e.g., IcyHot) can offer a great complement to cannabis-based products.

✓ Do stay consistent.

Try to stick with a cannabis routine for at least 30 days and explore journaling about your doses to refine your best practices.

✗ Don't be afraid to get high.

Many people who use cannabis for pain report other mental health benefits.

✓ Do use full-spectrum CBD for pain if you don't want to get high (or can't because of your responsibilities).

Remember that full-spectrum CBD contains small and trace amounts of THC. The cannabinoids work better together, so full-spectrum is the more effective option.

✓ Do always be honest with your doctor or pain specialist when using cannabis for pain.

Note that cannabis can have interactions with other drugs and can also affect your tolerance to anesthesia. So remember that honesty with your doctor is always the best policy.

Frequently Asked Questions, Answered

Q I have chronic pain. I spoke to my doctor about using cannabis; they were supportive but didn't have experience. Are there cannabis-specific doctors?

A A new and growing field of medicine is doctors who specialize in cannabis. High-profile examples include the Knox Docs, an Oregon-based family of physicians who founded the American Cannabinoid Clinics, which provide specialized integrative cannabinoid care. There's Dr. Bonni Goldstein, medical director of Canna-Centers, who educates patients on the use of cannabis therapy. And there's the Advanced Integrative Medical Science Institute (AIMS Institute), which specializes in a number of modalities. Check the Resources section (page 139) for help finding a doctor.

Q I am having back pain and muscle spasms. How would you approach this with cannabis?

A I would take a two-delivery-method approach: an oral dose of cannabis and a topical cannabis product applied to the affected area. Look for a 1:1 ratio of THC to CBD for the best results.

Q I am currently on opioids for pain management associated with cancer. Can I still use cannabis?

A Yes, you can. Of course, consult your doctor first. But generally, opioids and cannabis work differently, through different systems in the body. So you can use them congruently. Based on the current science and data, I encourage those using opioids to use cannabis as well. Research has found that people using medical cannabis in conjunction with opioids have significant improvements in pain control with reduced doses of opioids, which leads to a lower risk of overdose and addiction. Many patients also report the cannabis aids with the side effects from opioids.

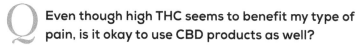

Q **Even though high THC seems to benefit my type of pain, is it okay to use CBD products as well?**

A I absolutely recommend that you use CBD along with your THC for pain. However, I do not recommend taking your pain meds, THC, and CBD all at the same time. Over the years, I have learned that timing out medication with THC can be vital. Using pharmaceuticals can bring relief in the short term, using THC can bring relief over time, and using CBD can help with the psychological effects of pain. So mind the time of your dose, and it can all work to your greatest benefit. Timing is always going to depend on the pain level and desired effect. Some people believe in dosing in intervals, 9 a.m., 12 p.m., 3 p.m., and 9 p.m., to keep their pain levels low. Others prefer to only dose when pain is present. There are many variables with the time of your dose. For example, are you trying to sleep? You will want to dose at least one hour before your desired bedtime.

Takeaways

- Remember that significant restrictions on cannabis research were only lifted a few years ago, but cannabis has been used for pain management for thousands of years. Every day the science is trickling in to show that cannabis can and will be a safer alternative to opioids for treating pain.

- When it comes to cannabis and pain, you have to stick with it. All cannabis use requires checking in with your body, knowing the most effective delivery method, and minding your effective dose.

- There's much discussion in the medical community about the way cannabis affects pain not just physically but mentally and emotionally. The mental undoubtedly affects the physical, and there is early evidence to suggest this is another promising way cannabis may benefit those in pain of all types.

CHAPTER 7

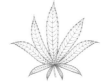

Beauty

CANNABIS HAS UNDENIABLY TAKEN THE MODERN beauty industry by storm, but cannabis as a beauty product has been around for thousands of years. At one of the birthplaces of Buddhism in Thailand, etchings have been found with instructions for using cannabis on the skin. Dry rubbing of cannabis leaves to treat horse wounds and oral delivery of cannabinoids for inflammation were practiced by the ancient Greeks.

Today cannabinoids, specifically CBD, have become major ingredients in beauty products. But do cannabinoids really serve a purpose when it comes to enhancing beauty? Mounting evidence shows CBD to have a host of benefits to the skin. As with other applications, the research is limited, but it has established that the skin is influenced by the endocannabinoid system. Receptors for the ECS have been identified in the skin, and cannabinoids have been receiving significant attention for their therapeutic potential for helping with various skin and cosmetic disorders. A growing body of clinical evidence suggests topical applications of CBD are effective for eczema, psoriasis, pruritus (severe itching), and other inflammatory skin conditions.

Your skin covers your entire body and is filled with cannabinoid receptors, so it's an incredible opportunity for cannabinoid exploration. Many of the issues and challenges relating to our skin are due to inflammation, and CBD is a known anti-inflammatory. So CBD beauty really does make sense. Of course, a CBD beauty product is only as good as its other ingredients and its potency (the amount of CBD and other cannabinoids in the product).

With the popularity of CBD beauty products came an explosion of gimmicky, and frankly useless, products. Why should you buy a CBD mascara when you don't have endocannabinoid receptors in your eyelashes? Another favorite trick of the beauty industry is to use hemp seed oil (also known as cannabis sativa seed oil) and pretend it could have the benefits of CBD. Hemp seed oil is a great ingredient in some respects, but it contains absolutely no cannabinoids or CBD. When navigating cannabis for beauty, it is important to always buy lab-tested products, so you know you're getting what you pay for. When researching products, check with the company or retailer to review lab tests.

With commercialization and legalization, we're even seeing THC-containing beauty products, from lotions to beauty tonics, and even transdermal makeup that gets you high. The ever-evolving world of cannabis beauty can bring so much into your life beyond just skin benefits. Transdermal products, like THC primer, can not only prime your skin and keep your makeup in place but also deliver a powerful dose of THC into your bloodstream. This can be a great option for those who have social anxiety before a big date or meeting. In this chapter, we'll explore the many ways to experience cannabis beauty, discuss what you should look for when buying a cannabis beauty product, and consider how to integrate these products into your routines.

What to Use

When it comes to cannabis beauty, CBD is the main player. CBD is a powerful antioxidant, which makes it a star ingredient for skincare. Also, CBD reduces inflammation, regulates oil production, and neutralizes free radical damage. It's recommended for those with inflamed and compromised skin, as well as sensitive and dry skin types. It can also benefit those with aging skin. CBD-based skincare can be used daily. It combines well with other active ingredients that calm and nourish the skin barrier, such as ceramides, hyaluronic acid, peptides, and niacinamides.

Be cautious with CBD skincare. Since it's an unregulated industry, and cannabinoid research in skincare and beauty is still limited, it's undetermined how CBD might interact with other active ingredients. We do not know what activates or deactivates CBD when it comes to other products. It's not recommended to use CBD skin products that contain alcohol, as this may counteract its beneficial effects and heighten some inflammatory skin conditions. Do you have skin allergies? Does your skin easily break out or react to certain carrier oils or other substances? Adding CBD to your skincare could create irritation. You do need to do your own research, check ingredient lists, and pay close attention to the results.

Lip balms and lip glosses containing both THC and CBD have popped up in hemp retailers and dispensaries alike. If you have dry, cracked lips, cold sores, or even lip pimples (ow!) a cannabis-infused lip product can really do wonders. If you are experiencing pain, full-spectrum CBD or THC will be a better option for lip care.

Cannabis beauty includes a vast world of body and personal care. Cannabis-infused body care such as bath bombs, bubble baths, lotions and bath salts can transform your personal wellness. Your skin is full of endocannabinoid receptors, and there's mounting evidence that integrating cannabinoids into your bath or shower can have serious benefits. Cannabis can play a huge role in improving circulation as well as softening and nourishing your skin. When you soak in a tub of cannabinoids, your skin absorbs the cannabinoids, and they penetrate deeply. Try a weekly cannabis-infused bath to experience the benefits. For those without tubs or time for soaking, transdermal shower gels are a powerful option for body care. And you can follow up your shower or bath with a cannabis-infused body lotion or salve.

Another amazing way to explore cannabis beauty is with hair care and scalp products. People are using cannabis-infused hair and scalp treatments to break through dermatological conditions like dandruff and scalp acne.

Pro Tips

✓ Do check the dose.

When it comes to cannabis beauty, dose and quality of product are the most important factors when making purchasing decisions. Topical products should have a dosage of at least 25 mg of CBD per serving. With topical applications, it's the opposite of oral cannabis: more is more. Trying higher-dose products—100 mg, 200 mg, or 1000 mg—will make the difference when it comes to approaching beauty.

✓ Do ask for COAs.

When evaluating your options, ask for lab tests (certificates of analysis, or COAs) for anything related to cannabis beauty (whether the product is from Sephora or a dispensary), to ensure the product is dosed correctly. You can request COAs directly from brands and retailers. Most reputable companies have them available in the footer of their websites.

✗ Don't confuse hemp seed oil with CBD.

Remember that hemp seed oil, or cannabis sativa seed oil, does not mean the product contains CBD. Don't be the victim of a CBD cash grab. You want to see CBD or hemp CBD extract listed in the ingredients.

✓ Do your own research on the brand.

Do your research into the brand, because reputation and transparency matters when buying CBD beauty products. Does the brand participate in legal cannabis markets? Do they have lab testing information visible on the website? Do they have sustainable and transparent business practices?

✓ Do stick with it.

Stick with cannabis beauty products for a minimum of 90 days before you decide they don't work.

✓ Do look for supplement panels and FDA disclosure.

The most legit CBD beauty products will have supplement panels and FDA disclosures on the packaging. Even though these products are unregulated, the best companies self-regulate and provide the consumer with all necessary information.

✓ Do check the net weight.

When it comes to CBD products, this is important because of dosing. What you are paying for is milligrams per gram. So understanding that the product is 16 total ounces, with 200 mg of CBD, will help you understand what you are getting for every serving. Companies often will have only 10 mg CBD in a product with a 6 oz. weight. This is useless for a consumer and why a product having a clear net weight is important. A clearly listed net weight is a signifier of a solid

CBD product. If the product doesn't list a net weight, I would avoid it.

✓ Do check the type of CBD.

Is the CBD full spectrum, broad spectrum, or isolate? This information not only helps you choose the product that meets your needs; transparency in the classification of the CBD extract is a sign of a trustworthy brand.

✓ Do check the label dates.

Look for a batch or manufacturing date on the product. Beauty products specifically have batch numbers, manufacturing date, and expiration dates on their labels. This is important not only because it's what reputable companies do, but because you want to avoid expired products.

✓ Do use CBD for hydration.

Whether on your skin or on your lips, lather up with a CBD beauty product. CBD has moisturizing properties that can help combat dehydration and dryness.

✗ Don't be afraid to stack products.

The beauty industry loves to bring us new products; thus there are countless cannabis beauty products available. Since most cannabis beauty products are topical, don't be afraid to stack them.

✓ Do try a cannabis spa experience.

From cannabis-infused manicures and pedicures (cannacures) to CBD-infused facials, exploring CBD and cannabis beauty in a spa setting is a must-do.

Frequently Asked Questions, Answered

Q Even though I don't have terrible acne, I do get random pimples sometimes that sprout up on my nose or my forehead. How can I use CBD or cannabis to help with this issue?

A You're in luck! There are many ways that cannabinoids can help with acne flare-ups. First, with an existing breakout, cannabis's anti-inflammatory properties will lessen redness and pain, as well as swelling, whether applied directly to the area or ingested. Also, THC's analgesic properties are very beneficial when it comes to the pain associated with severe acne. Next, many cannabinoids, but especially CBG and CBGA (cannabigerolic acid), have been shown to have very strong antimicrobial and antibacterial properties. What does this mean? Well, the bacteria that caused the acne in the first place will be killed when it comes into contact with these powerful cannabinoids. Don't worry if you can't find many CBG-based topical or beauty products; CBD and THC are also known to have potent antibacterial effects. Another way cannabis can help with acne is by reducing stress, potentially preventing acne before it appears or lessening its duration. Acne is known to have a strong correlation with our stress levels, so anything you can do to reduce stress can and will help alleviate many of these issues.

Q Will a cannabis beauty product get me high if it contains a lot of THC?

A In almost every circumstance, the answer is no; even high-THC cannabis-infused products will not cross into the bloodstream. However, if a product uses true nanotechnology or describes itself as transdermal, then it is possible to get high from a beauty product. Depending on what you're looking for, this can be a huge positive or a turnoff. The lesson here is that you should always do your research, ask for lab tests, and read the label and packaging carefully before purchasing or using any products—and especially before assuming that they will or won't have a psychoactive effect.

Q I tried a cannabis skincare product, and it made me break out/gave me a rash/made my issue worse! Did I react this way because of the CBD/cannabinoids in the product?

A More often than not, this type of reaction is caused by other active or inactive ingredients used in the product. Just as with conventional beauty products, you have to find what works for you and your skin. Generally if you take a look at the labeling of most beauty products, you'll find dozens of ingredients, likely including many that you cannot pronounce and don't know anything about. Many of us have undiagnosed allergies to cosmetic ingredients, so I encourage you to compare the cannabis product's full ingredient list with some of your favorite beauty products. If you find any ingredients that you have not been exposed to before, research and see whether any of these ingredients can potentially cause these types of reactions. Skincare is complex, and all you can do is educate yourself and be empowered by the knowledge that you gain through experience. Be open-minded, but if your skin gets red or reacts badly, it is telling you to stop!

Takeaways

- When buying CBD beauty products, look for CBD in the ingredients or formula. Other acceptable terms include hemp CBD, full-spectrum hemp extract, phytocannabinoid-rich hemp oil, and hemp extract.

- Think logically about the product and the way it delivers cannabinoids to the endocannabinoid system. Does the area to which you will apply the product have cannabinoid receptors?

- Combine delivery methods in your CBD beauty products for maximum results. For example, you might start your day with a CBD tincture, follow it up with a CBD-infused primer under your makeup (for preventing breakouts under your makeup), then end your night with a CBD shower gel and a CBD eye cream.

- Itching, dry skin, redness, and inflammation are all proven to benefit from CBD skincare and beauty products.

- Not all CBD beauty products are created equal. Ask for lab tests before you buy the product.

CHAPTER 8

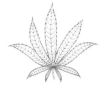

At the Gym

ACCORDING TO *MEN'S JOURNAL*, BASED ON A NEW study out of University of Colorado Boulder, nearly 82 percent of people who use legal cannabis consume before or after exercise (most often both), because it makes their workout more enjoyable and helps with a faster recovery. THC and CBD, the main active compounds found in the cannabis plant, have anti-inflammatory, muscle-relaxing, and pain-relieving effects, which can alleviate muscle soreness, muscle spasms, and arthritic joint pain. Cannabis doesn't make us invincible, but it does make us feel better faster.

You may be confused by a connection between exercise and cannabis because you've heard so much about the lazy stoner stereotype. But cannabinoids are actually the source for the famous "runner's high," the exhilaration that can come from intense exercise. Hormones called *endorphins* used to get the credit, but recent science shows that this feeling is actually activated by the endocannabinoid receptors connected to the reward pathways in the brain.

Too much THC can have side effects, so low doses are better for exercise. Most people who use cannabis for fitness suggest not overindulging before a workout, because it can impair focus and performance. In extreme cases, if you are too high, this could lead to injury. So it's important to be mindful that less is more with cannabis and fitness. A popular approach for those looking to maximize their workouts with cannabis is microdosing. Taking a small amount of cannabis, like 1 or 2 mg as an edible, seems to be a great approach for exercise, because it can tone down racing thoughts and decrease inflammation.

One thing it seems everyone agrees on when it comes to cannabis and fitness is the role of CBD. Mounting evidence suggests that you should take CBD as soon as possible after workouts for better recovery. Preliminary research suggests that this can reduce general pain, muscle spasms, stiffness, and inflammation. There is also scientific data to support the idea that CBD reduces some of the inflammation-promoting proteins specifically released during exercise. By following up your workout with CBD you can recover faster and reduce inflammation.

What to Use

When it comes to using cannabis for fitness, there are two main categories of use: before the workout and after. Remember that using cannabis while you exercise can be dangerous. When it comes to before your workout, strain selection will be extremely important. Finding hybrid or sativa strains that agree with you will maximize your performance. Avoiding indica strains, or strains that give you a body high, is recommended. The top strains for fitness are Sour

Diesel, Jack Herer, Durban Poison, Super Lemon Haze, Sour Cheese, and Purple Haze.

As for using cannabis before a workout, I recommend avoiding smoking. Tinctures, vapes, microdose edibles, microdose beverages, and topicals are all better options. Finding your perfect dose will be key, because with fitness you are truly looking for your sweet spot—feeling like you're elevated, and your performance is enhanced, but you're not completely high. Once you find it, you will feel it. If you feel too sleepy, tired, or hungry, you are far past the sweet spot.

In chapter 4, when we discussed the munchies (page 57), we explored THCV. It's a minor cannabinoid perfect for those looking for a cannabinoid that can increase focus and performance. It's important to remember that if you smoke or consume too much delta-9-THC with THCV, it's not guaranteed to work.

When it comes to the post-workout cannabis application, you have a wide variety of products and experiences available. Remember that CBD is the anti-inflammatory molecule, so choose products that have both THC and CBD. Ratios and full-spectrum CBD products will work more effectively than pure CBD products. Of all the available information on cannabis post-workout, there is a general consensus that you should consume CBD as soon as possible after a workout. This could be a tincture, a gummy, or even smoking a high-CBD strain like ACDC. Patricia Frye, chief medical officer at cannabis education startup HelloMD, has been quoted as saying, "Athletes may be able to return to intense workouts faster because they feel better faster."

For sore muscles and body recovery, there's a wide variety of pain lotions, creams, roll-ons, and salves. Remember when shopping that transdermals will be more effective, but they will also be more expensive. Either way, integrate these products into your routine post-shower. Your pores will be open, and it will maximize the benefits of the cannabis.

For injuries or extreme recovery (triathlons, marathons, etc.) look for high-dose pain products. From tinctures to topicals, you have a wide range of high-dose products to choose from.

Pro Tips

✘ Don't use cannabis for exercise if . . .

People who get anxious while high or who have heart conditions should abstain from cannabis use while exercising.

✘ Don't be too high in the gym.

Always be mindful that being too high in a gym or fitness studio can be dangerous, especially if you are working with heavy exercise equipment.

✓ Do explore dose and delivery method.

Play with ratios and mixing delivery methods. When it comes to fitness, I often love a blend of cannabinoids like CBG and THC. I will also mix the ways I consume it. For example, I will take a CBG gummy and vape THC before my workout.

✓ Do journal and track your workouts.

Journaling and tracking your cannabis consumption and your workouts can help you find your sweet spot. By noticing patterns and documenting desired effects, you can come up with a routine that meets your needs.

✓ Do use cannabis topicals before and after.

Always engage with cannabis topicals for body pain and soreness, both before and after exercising.

✓ Do recover with CBD.

Consider adding CBD to your post-workout routine or gym shower to help speed up your recovery.

✓ Do explore roll-ons.

Roll-on topicals are better options than salves or balms, because they are easier to apply if you are mid-workout or on a long hike.

✓ Do hydrate.

Hydration is key when consuming cannabis and incredibly important when you are using cannabis while you work out, since dry mouth is a side effect of cannabis use. Make sure to load up on water for hydration when using cannabis with any kind of physical activity.

✓ Do be mindful of edibles.

Avoid edibles when it comes to fitness because of their time delay. It's often more challenging to get the timing right when using edibles as a delivery method.

Frequently Asked Questions, Answered

Q I am now using cannabis and CBD daily, but I have never tried to integrate it into my workouts. What's the best first step?

A Since you're new to combining cannabis with your gym routine, start slow with CBD. Since CBD is nonimpairing, you will stay sober while enjoying its anti-inflammatory effects for post-workout recovery. CBD can also put you in a calm, focused state of mind that can be helpful for more intense cardio sessions or heavy weight lifting. If you're a yoga practitioner, CBD may be very beneficial when it comes to getting into the right mindset for your session. If you find you're comfortable with a little THC, I recommend a microdose, only 1 or 2 mg of an edible to start, or a few puffs on a joint. This can have a wonderful motivating effect that may get you into a great flow state, improving your focus on your muscles' reactions to certain movements and your awareness of your heart rate and breathing patterns.

Definitely don't overdo it; you don't want to end up with anxiety from too much THC combined with an elevated heart rate from working out. Another beneficial molecule in my experience is THCV. It provides a strong but clear, focused energy (with the added benefit of appetite suppression) that I often prefer to caffeine, especially before a cardio-heavy workout.

Q **I am super sore from a long run/leg day. What products should I choose to help me recover and alleviate the pain and soreness?**

A Ah, that infamous day-after soreness! The good news is that you have options. My first suggestion would be a higher-dose (preferably full-spectrum) CBD bath bomb. The hot water as well as the dose of cannabinoids will really help your muscles relax. After that, I would lather my legs up with the most effective cannabis topical I could find. Ideally you would use a product that combines other pain-relieving and inflammation-reducing ingredients with cannabis in an effective formulation. After that, you can choose to light up, eat a bit of an edible, or try a tincture. I know you're in pain, but still, you do not want to dose yourself with THC past what you can tolerate. You may find that the more pain you're in, the higher a dose you can tolerate, but start low and go slow, and you will be on the road to recovery in no time.

Q **I smoked some THC flower before going on a run, but it seemed like as soon as I got going, the high went away. What happened, and what can I do to avoid this?**

A I have definitely noticed that during intense workouts or other experiences when adrenaline may be coming into play, it's common to feel that your high can be dampened or perhaps completely negated. One way you can counteract this is with edible THC. Since edible THC has an inherently longer duration of effect, this may be a great strategy to have your high last longer through your session. I've also noticed that combining THC flower or concentrate consumption with full-spectrum CBD can give a more resilient effect, since there are so many other cannabinoids at play. This comes down to the entourage effect, and you may also find you have a more balanced, enjoyable experience as well.

Takeaways

- Runner's high isn't caused by endorphins; it's an effect of the endocannabinoid system.

- Explore both pre- and post-workout cannabis consumption. Trying both can often lead to finding what works best for you.

- Start low and go slow is always the best approach.

- Never put yourself in danger, and always be mindful of being too high in a gym or around heavy exercise equipment.

- THC is great for pain management and injury recovery.

- CBD is great for inflammation and recovery.

CHAPTER 9

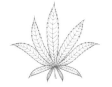

Between the Sheets

BACK WHEN I FIRST WAS A BUDTENDER, THE thing that shocked me the most about working in cannabis was how few people came to buy weed just to get high—because getting high was all I had ever been taught about the plant. Understanding the power cannabis was having in the bedroom for people is what truly blew my mind, and it might do the same for you. Cannabis can transform your experience of both sleep and sex, thanks to the integral role that the endocannabinoid system plays in our bodies. We'll explore both of those topics in this chapter.

In this chapter we'll explore how cannabis can treat insomnia for those who struggle with sleep issues. Cannabinoids can aid in your overall wellness by helping you get a better night's rest. The endocannabinoid system plays a pivotal role in our sleep, which is why cannabis is such an effective tool for this. Now there are even newly discovered molecules like CBN (cannabinol), which has growing anecdotal support as "the sleep cannabinoid."

As with other uses, more medical research is needed to fully understand the role that cannabis has in regard to sleep and sleep disorders. Research into cannabis and insomnia shows that CBD may have therapeutic potential for the treatment of insomnia. New research on synthetic cannabinoids like nabilone and dronabinol shows that they have short-term benefits for sleep apnea. CBD may additionally hold promise for REM sleep behavior disorder (a condition in which people physically act out their dreams) and excessive daytime sleepiness.

Cannabis is an aphrodisiac and has many different applications for sex: boosting libido, decreasing anxiety during sex, helping with painful sex, enhancing touch. In one recent study, 68 percent of women said sex was more pleasurable after using cannabis. From finding the right strains to considering the new, innovative sex products you may find when visiting a dispensary, we will dive into all things cannabis and sex.

What to Use

Cannabis is an effective sleep aid for many, as it can slow the mind, relax the body, and dissolve pain to help you fall and stay asleep. THC is often the most effective choice for good sleeping, even though many people find full-spectrum CBD to be capable of putting them to sleep. I encourage you to choose nonsmokable delivery options like tinctures, capsules, vapes, and edibles, which are more known for keeping people asleep for longer. Also, smoking can be hard on the lungs if you need cannabis daily or frequently to sleep. When it comes to strains, hybrids and indicas are best. Sativas can induce more energy and anxiety, so it's best to avoid them if your aim is to improve your sleep quality. Taking hot baths has proven scientific benefits for improving sleep, and cannabis-infused baths are another insider tip for using cannabis to improve your sleep.

When you're not looking for a good night's sleep, cannabis can enhance your sex life in multiple ways, from increasing sensitivity and pleasure to decreasing pain. It can lower inhibition, allowing a deeper level of intimacy or connection. For some, puffing on a joint of the right strain is the perfect pre-sex delivery method. For others, nonsmoking modern products like lubricants, oils, tinctures, and microdosed edibles are better suited. As with all cannabis, everyone's body and experience will vary. In a vast majority of the anecdotal evidence I've explored, the consensus is that less is more when it comes to consuming cannabis for sex. Remember that if you choose to smoke or inhale cannabis, it may give you dry mouth. So have water nearby!

For Insomnia

The biggest challenge to using cannabis for sleep is going to be finding the right dose, which will take some trial and error. You may also need to combine delivery methods. For example, you may need to vape a high-THC strain like Tahoe OG Kush to get to sleep fast, and take a 10 mg 1:1 THC/CBD capsule to stay asleep. The key is to find the right combination and dose that helps you fall asleep, stay asleep, and not have a hangover in the morning. Sleep-specific strains for insomnia include Tahoe OG Kush, Sweet and Sour Widow, Skywalker OG, and Northern Lights.

CBN, or cannabinol, is a mildly psychoactive component found in cannabis that is now used and available in many forms as a sleep aid or sedative. This cannabinoid has become notorious for helping people achieve the best sleep of their lives. The dispensary will most likely have a small selection of CBN products. You can also find a number of hemp-derived CBN products available online.

For Boosting Libido

You can use libido-boosting cannabis strains like Green Crack, Grandaddy Purple, and Do-Si-Dos. More modern products like lubricants and arousal oils can also boost libido in the bedroom. Most of these topical products are applied to the genitals to increase blood flow and circulation to the area.

For Anxiety during Sex

Top strains for anxiety in the bedroom are Bubba Kush, Skywalker OG, Blueberry Lambsbread, and Kosher Kush. If you are uninterested in smoking before sex, you could also try a high-CBD tincture for pre-sex anxiety. For a topical-only approach, consider a hot bath with a cannabis-infused bath bomb before sex. Then follow up with a high-CBD lubricant, the perfect product for sex-related anxiety.

For Pain during Sex

Lubes, oils, and suppositories are all staples of most dispensaries that can aid in painful sex. When dealing with painful sex, you want to use a product with higher THC content than CBD. Ratioed products are a great choice, but you may find that CBD-only will not be enough to manage pain.

If you are choosing a smokable, look for strains with terpenes that may ease pain, such as beta-caryophyllene, humulene, myrcene, and caryophyllene. Strains like Zkittlez, G13, Cannatonic, and Harlequin are all great strains for pain relief during sex.

For Enhancing Touch

Many seasoned cannabis users will tell you that certain strains increase sensitivity to touch and change sensations for the better. Everyone is different, so some strains may enhance touch for you, while your partner may respond better to different strains. Strains like ACDC give you a rich terpene profile and strong CBD:THC ratio. Other strains to ramp up erogenous play are Bubblegum Kush, Sour Diesel, and Jillybean.

Cannabis-infused massage oils are also a great addition to foreplay.

Pro Tips

✓ Do adjust your dose if you're still high in the morning.

Do not give up on finding the right dose for sleep. If you are still high the next day or experiencing a hangover type of feeling, you need to dial your dose back.

✓ Do explore CBN for sleep.

Look for products with CBN (cannabinol), a.k.a. the sleep molecule, for better sleep. Ask your budtender for CBN products or check COAs (certificates of analysis) for a product's cannabinoid profile.

✓ Do pay attention to the ingredients . . . cannabis lubes are not all equal.

It is incredibly important when choosing a cannabis lube that you pay attention to the ingredients. Not just because your genitals are extremely sensitive, but because some cannabis lubes are not latex safe; oil-based lubes do not work with condoms. For those looking for a latex-safe cannabis lube, make sure to check that the product is water-based. This is also something to keep in mind when you are choosing products to use with toys. Some toys will require silicone or water-based lubricants, so mind the ingredients as you select a product.

✗ Don't use cannabis lubricants or oils only for intercourse.

I have sold cannabis lubes for nearly six and a half years, and the biggest thing I hear is how many people use cannabis lubes and oils for more than intercourse. Self-pleasure and reducing pain are two reasons why people use cannabis lubricants and oils.

✓ Do take cannabis baths for sleep and for sex.

Cannabis-infused baths combined with essential oils can make a significant impact in the bedroom. Choosing a bath bomb, bath salt, or bubble bath infused with cannabis can help you get a significant improvement in your sleep. A hot cannabis bath before sex can also help you relax deeper into your body.

✓ Don't indulge in high doses of THC before sex.

High doses of THC will diminish your sex drive and put you to sleep. Remember low and moderate doses are where cannabis is proven to heighten sexual climax. A micro dose is 1 to 2.5 mg, a low dose is 2.5 to 5 mg, and a moderate dose is 5 to 10 mg. Anything over 10 mg is considered a high dose.

✓ Do use cannabis to get comfortable with your body.

A significant number of people, especially women, struggle with being comfortable with their bodies when it comes to sex. Those with sexual trauma or who struggle with gender identity often face especially difficult inhibitions with relaxing into their body when it comes to sex. Using cannabis can help relax you and keep you out of your head, which can lead to more enjoyable and less anxious sex.

Frequently Asked Questions, Answered

Q I am having some success with my insomnia in terms of falling asleep, but staying asleep seems to be harder to treat. What type of dosing schedule or strategy should I use in order to not wake up after three to four hours?

A Insomnia is always challenging to successfully manage with any medication, cannabis included. But fear not! Here are some ways you can find relief First, make sure you are taking a strong enough dose of the product/cannabinoid you are using. For example, if you are using full-spectrum CBD, I would recommend you try to double your regular daytime dose (or perhaps triple it, if a double dose isn't strong enough). Also, ingestibles will generally offer a longer duration of effect that can keep you asleep longer. A strategy I have used before is smoking a little bit of THC flower before bed to get me sleepy, then right when I'm already in bed, swallowing a 11 THC CBD capsule. That way, you give yourself the best chance to slowly digest the capsule once you're already asleep.

Q My partner and I tried smoking some cannabis before sex, but the effect was not exactly as intended. We both became a bit anxious and had dry mouths, and it took us a while to be able to calm down and get in the mood. What did we do wrong?

A This happens very often; don't worry. It is possible the strain was not compatible with your body chemistry or was not ideal as a pre-sex choice. Dosage can also make a huge impact in some of these side effects. With sex, the general rule of thumb is to consume a bit less than you would before any other activity, until you know how the specific strain or product will interact with your and your partner's sexual performance. Sometimes THC can raise our heart rate, which can have a negative effect on our state of mind, taking us out of the "zone" and even causing anxiety. If you want a low-risk option, try some CBD instead. You can find some great hemp flower or a high-CBD strain to substitute for your regular THC-laden cannabis strains. Just remember, stay calm, be nonjudgmental, and don't try to rush things if you aren't feeling comfortable. Sex is very personal, and cannabis can enhance our connection to ourselves and others, but sometimes that enhancement can feel overwhelming. I'll say it again start low and go slow!

Q **I want to try a cannabis lube, but I need to ensure it's safe for use with latex condoms. What should I look for in a product?**

A The first thing you should look for is that the lube is advertised as being water-based. Then look at the ingredients list and ensure water (or an ingredient that is water-based, like aloe) is the first ingredient. Coconut oil, olive oil, any oil really, should be an immediate red flag, as oil can degrade latex, rendering it ineffective. Next, you may want to look for a product that is using a verified nanotechnology, rather than a simple "water-soluble" formulation (you can request this information directly from the brand). Many of those formulations use sugar or starch-based ingredients that can and will cause infections down there (sugar feeds bacteria!). Always be cautious when it comes to your intimate areas, and do your research before diving in.

Takeaways

- Finding the right dose for the bedroom will be the most challenging part of your cannabis journey. From sleep to sex, cannabis use in the bedroom is all about figuring out the best dose.

- If you are experiencing hangover symptoms or you are still high the next day, you're using too much cannabis.

- Practice makes perfect. Consider testing products and strains before you do the deed or bring them into the bedroom with a partner.

- Explore nonsmokable delivery methods for the bedroom.

CHAPTER 10

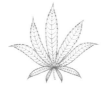

For Aging Gracefully

CANNABIS IS A POWERFUL TOOL WHEN IT COMES to staying healthy as we age, because of its antioxidant, anti-aging molecular properties. There's notable evidence mounting that the use of cannabis can counter and influence the effects of aging in many different ways. In this chapter, we will explore and discuss how both THC and CBD can help us deal with our aging brain, sore joints and bones, and menopause.

Even with my life dedicated to cannabis and my extensive knowledge, I'm surprised at how much positive, important, and promising research there is when it comes to cannabis and aging. Yes, aging comes with the decline of our bones, joints, and muscles. This weakening of our bodies, combined with inflammation, can bring significant pain. Feeding the powerhouse that is the endocannabinoid system and tapping into the anti-inflammatory capacity of cannabis molecules can aid in the pain and discomfort that comes with aging. Whatever your concerns about your health, quality of life, and overall wellness as you age, there are so many possibilities to explore for using cannabis to age gracefully.

In previous chapters, you've seen how cannabis can aid with sleep, mood, appetite, and pain, all of which can become concerns as we age. But cannabis can do a lot more than just treat the symptoms. For example, one fact of age is the slowing or stoppage of the body's lipid production, leading to dry skin. The endocannabinoid system includes endogenous lipid mediators that are present in nearly all tissues and may be responsible for producing lipids.

Cannabis may altogether reverse some aspects of the aging process altogether. A recent study from the University of Bonn, in partnership with the Hebrew University of Jerusalem, found that cannabis seems to undo the aging process in the brains of mice. In the study, when mice were given small doses of THC, "it looked as though the THC treatment turned back the molecular clock," according to the study director. As *Scientific American* summarized the results, "after the elderly animals were given THC, their performances improved to the point that they resembled those of young, untreated mice."

Countless other studies are available that conclude cannabinoids are able to improve the efficiency of the body's mitochondria, the powerhouse of the cell. And researchers have found that cannabinoids can remove harmful molecules from the tissue of the brain and central nervous system, increasing brain activity and mitigating the aging process.

Overall, there is a strong case for the cannabis plant bringing us its anti-aging benefits.

What to Use

Unlocking the promise of cannabis when it comes to aging, as with all cannabis use, isn't just about understanding why to use but also *how*. You can smoke cannabis or vape it, but for aging, there are much more effective delivery methods and approaches.

In my experience, the best practice for anti-aging benefits is to create a regimen or routine with twice-daily oral cannabinoids and topicals. When you look at the science around aging, cannabis, perimenopause, and menopause, it's clear that topical and ingestible cannabinoids can make an impact.

Oral cannabinoids taken daily, dosed in the morning and evening, are best for managing the effects of aging. Since the dose duration is significantly lengthened, dosing in the morning and again in the evening will keep the cannabinoids flowing through your bloodstream, allowing your body a constant supply of these beneficial molecules. Consider tinctures, capsules, and edibles the best delivery methods. Pairing the daily oral dose with topicals from salves, bath bombs, lotions, and oils will help your aging skin. Combining both delivery methods with consistency is key to getting results.

When it comes to aging, strain is not as important as it is with managing sleep issues. Instead, when approaching cannabis for aging, we need to look at the cannabinoids specifically and the cannabinoid profile of the product. A full-spectrum CBD tincture or a ratio product that contains THC, CBD, and the full cannabinoid profile is key. CBD-isolate products or products without the full-spectrum profile won't bring you the lipids, phytocannabinoids, or terpenes that are also important for anti-aging benefits. The strain itself does not appear to be a significant factor in any of my research. Avoid broad-spectrum and CBD-isolate products, and reach for full-spectrum options.

Another major factor to consider in selecting products is dose. You may need to explore with some trial and error. When calculating your dose, consider your height and weight. Additionally, consider your current pain levels and stress. If you are experiencing joint or muscle pain, start your dose higher. If you are not in pain and just looking to tap into cannabinoids' anti-aging properties, you can start your dose lower. A micro dose is 1 to 2.5 mg, a low dose is 2.5 to 5 mg, and a moderate dose is 5 to 10 mg. Anything over 10 mg is considered a high dose.

Over the years, I have noticed cannabis can affect me differently depending on what time of the month it is and where I am in my cycle. Just as with other applications, listening to your body is key. Our fluctuating hormones can affect the high in many ways; sometimes I will feel significantly more high and sensitive with my usual dose. Other times, I don't feel high or any effects at all, and I need more. Remember, your body is incredibly sensitive, and our endocannabinoid system is unique to each of us. Listen to your body and adjust your dose accordingly. Don't be afraid of topicals with high doses like 250 or 1000 mg; your body will love it. Remember that transdermal topicals may be more effective and work faster, but they could get you high. Balms, salves, bath bombs, bath salts, bubble baths, and oil-based products won't get you high.

I know I may sound like a broken record, but this is important: you've really gotta stick with the routine you build. The most impact from cannabis is not experienced by taking it when you're actively having hot flashes or a mood swing. It's by reaching for these magic molecules daily, to nourish your endocannabinoid system and create equilibrium in your body. Pay attention to your body, stick with your routine, adjust as needed, and let the plant heal you from the inside out.

Pro Tips

✓ **Do use cannabis for sleep and mood.**

Review previous chapters, because sleep and mood disruptions are common symptoms that happen as we age, and cannabis can help.

✓ **Do use cannabis suppositories, oils, and lubes for vaginal dryness.**

In chapter 7, we discussed how cannabis is hydrating for the skin. There are so many great products from topicals to transdermals that can help with age-related vaginal dryness. If you are lucky enough to find suppositories at your dispensary, you won't be disappointed.

✓ **Do explore ratios with both THC and CBD.**

In all my research, I've found that both THC and CBD have a significant impact for women in perimenopause and menopause. THC is a great molecule because among other things, it can lower body temperature. CBD has significant impact on hot flashes and night sweats; it's known to influence the body's production of serotonin, the key hormone that stabilizes our mood, happiness, and feelings of wellbeing.

✓ **Do track your symptoms and cannabis use.**

Keep a record of the intensity of your symptoms, along with what you're doing for them and what else is going on in your life. After a few entries, look for patterns and experiment with your dosing, delivery systems, and time of consumption.

✓ **Do be cautious with high-THC strains and products.**

We know high THC can be great for pain but be mindful of your dose. Long-term use of high-THC products can cause further disruption in mood and sleep and increased depression.

✓ Do choose full-spectrum products.

Isolates and broad-spectrum products are better than nothing, but when it comes to menopause, the full cannabinoid profile and entourage effect have been seen as notably more effective.

✓ Do infuse your own products.

While some dispensaries may cater to women or clients looking for vaginal serums, others may not. Do not be discouraged. Find an oil or serum you love and infuse it yourself. You want to get estrogen flowing to the pelvic region, which will deliver fresh oxygen to the urinary tract tissues and sexual organs. This keeps you elastic and healthy. Since cannabinoids are a vasodilator, they can increase blood flow to the region. The topical application of cannabinoids to the area can also relax muscles, calm pain-perceiving nerves, and fight inflammation. You can see how integral a product infused with cannabis could be to this area, so if you can't find it . . . MAKE YOUR OWN! You'll find instructions for this in the next chapter.

✓ Do take oral cannabinoids.

As mentioned, there are countless studies that point to cannabinoids' ability to improve mitochondrial function. On a molecular level, cannabis regulates mitochondrial activity, acting as an antioxidant and helping clear harmful molecules from the brain and the nervous system. This process is believed to reduce the aging process and play a role in increasing brain function. So taking oral cannabinoids daily—tinctures, edibles, capsules, and oils—can also ease the aging process from the inside out. I suggest a minimum of 50 mg of full-spectrum CBD daily.

Frequently Asked Questions, Answered

Q My hot flashes come on quick and unexpectedly. Is there anything you recommend that could work quickly?

A Many products in dispensaries now have nanotechnology for quick-onset effects. When choosing edibles or tinctures to manage hot flashes, look for products labeled "rapid onset" or nanotechnology. These will work much more quickly than traditional products. Other products to seek are sublinguals, which will distribute the cannabinoids differently than traditional edibles.

Q Sometimes my menopause symptoms occur while I'm at work. Is there anything you recommend for discretion?

A In the past few years, there has been a significant proliferation of cannabis-infused patches. If you're in the workplace, it's important to mind your dose, but a high-CBD patch can deliver cannabinoids easily while you work, with complete discretion.

Q I can't seem to manage my weight since going into menopause. How can I get the benefits of THC without creating the munchies, which will only further exacerbate my weight issues?

A When you're needing to monitor your weight because of menopause, there are many things you can do. First, avoid heavy indica strains, which normally induce the munchies. Seek out THCV or high-THCV strains, like Durban Poison and Jack Herer. In a study published in 2015, cannabis use was statistically associated with a lower body mass index and a lower percentage of fat mass. So, generally cannabis use does not seem to cause weight gain. You may just want to switch the strain or explore other minor cannabinoids.

Menopause has really taken my sex drive away. Can cannabis help?

According to research, cannabis users have 20 percent more sex. I recommend exploring a cannabinoid product with essential oils or other ingredients that stimulate sex drive. In my experience the entourage effect or products with other aphrodisiacs (like the herb horny goat weed, a.k.a. barrenwort) can be extremely effective when combined with cannabis.

How do I develop a routine with cannabis for menopause?

I've spoken to countless women in menopause who actively use cannabis for menopause symptoms. They all had developed their own routines for constantly using cannabis. The constant delivery of cannabinoids helped them manage their symptoms. Most used not just a single product but multiples. All of them used tinctures daily, morning and night, to deliver different dosages of cannabis. Many used edibles for sleep, and some preferred CBN to traditional THC. Last, almost all the women I interviewed used vaginal applications of cannabinoids. Some women preferred oil-based to water-based products. Overall, their best advice was to gather an arsenal of products in your medicine cabinet to constantly tackle menopause symptoms.

Takeaways

- Do not be afraid to put cannabis directly on the vagina, vulva, or inside your body. The closer the cannabis is to the area where it's needed, the more effective it may be.

- Combine both THC and CBD into a routine and stick with it. Indulge in both oral and topical cannabinoids for the best results.

- Share your experiences or build community in a support group. Finding the right dose or ritual could be aided by having community support or someone to talk to who is also experiencing menopause.

- Explore minor cannabinoids like CBG, THCV, and CBDA, to see whether they bring you relief outside of THC and CBD.

- Cannabis is a great alternative for aches, pains, joint issues, and inflammation that come with aging.

- Cannabis doesn't just help us age with ease; science shows it can actually have neuroprotective qualities and protect our brains from aging.

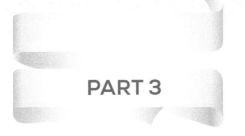

PART 3

FUN AND FOUNDATIONAL CANNABIS RECIPES

I'VE ENJOYED THE PRIVILEGE OF having supportive parents who came out of the cannabis closet with me 15 years ago. We have often spent time in the kitchen creating cannabis recipes and products together. Try it and you'll find that cooking with cannabis will deepen your connection to the plant. To get you started, I have included our family cannabis recipes in this section of the book, including the OG Kush Queen bath bomb recipe that started it all.

NEED-TO-KNOWS

There's a myriad of things that you can infuse with cannabis, from the basics like infusing butter and oil (your ticket to infusing almost anything) to making beauty products of your own. Having a basic level of cannabis infusion know-how can help you entertain with cannabis or engage in self-care. And in today's world of commercialized cannabis, it can also help you save a little money.

You can toss canna-butter (cannabis-infused butter) onto anything, from bread to a steak. You can infuse canna-oil into a smoothie or rub it on your skin. Once you master oil and butter infusions, the world is your cannabis oyster.

When you make your own products, you have more control over your dose. Maybe you want to customize your recipe with a high dose or a microdose. Calibrating a dose will be dependent on the potency of your cannabis flower or oil. If you buy from a licensed retailer, the potency should be listed on the product label. If you do not have the potency info, the rule of thumb is to assume the product is 15 percent potency. THC degrades at high heat, so mind your temps when cooking with cannabis. You should never exceed 340°F/171°C, because it will degrade the cannabis.

When making your own cannabis products, label everything. There is nothing scarier than finding rogue unlabeled weed brownies in a fridge, or your unlabeled gummies falling into the wrong hands.

Decarboxylation: Activating the Cannabinoids

Many cooks roast or toast their spices and herbs. When it comes to cooking or making products with cannabis, we do this, too. This is a process called decarboxylation, or decarbing, and it's how you activate the cannabis. Otherwise, it will not work.

Decarboxylation is a very aromatic process. Baking in a turkey roasting bag can assist with the smell, but I recommend just opening a window or doing this in a space with ventilation.

How to Decarb Cannabis:

1. Preheat the oven to 240°F/116°C.

2. Break up the cannabis flowers and buds into smaller pieces with your hands.

3. Place the cannabis in a single layer on a rimmed baking sheet.

4. Bake the cannabis for 40 minutes. Stir and mix while baking so that it cooks evenly.

5. When the cannabis is a darker color, a medium brown, and has dried out, remove the baking sheet from the oven and allow the cannabis to cool. The texture will be crumbly.

6. In a food processor, pulse the cannabis until it is coarsely ground. Place it in a mason jar with a lid and label it as decarboxylated flower. Store in a cool, dark place.

Must-Have Equipment

You'll need some simple kitchen gear for your cannabis cooking, some of which you may already have. You don't need to reserve specific kitchen tools as cannabis-only, as long as you wash them before re-using.

- Alcohol or alcohol wipes (for cleaning cannabis oil and residues)
- Baking sheets
- Bowls
- Cheesecloth
- Glass storage jars
- Gloves (your hands can get sticky from handling cannabis)
- Kitchen scale
- Slow cooker (e.g., a Crockpot)
- Spatulas

KEEP IN MIND

Cannabis and cannabis oil can be very sticky. So there can be a lot of sticky residue left after a recipe, as with making candy. Make sure to keep alcohol or alcohol wipes nearby; this will be your best friend when cleaning up cannabis oil and residue.

Cooking or making products with cannabis is NOT discreet. Well, cooking any of these recipes, or with cannabis in general, is going to be very fragrant. So if you are trying to be low-key or discreet, understand this is not the activity for you. If you are concerned about the smell, make sure to open all windows, turn on your kitchen vent, and have added ventilation.

Slow Cooker Canna-Butter

Yield: 2 cups **Prep time:** Varies

This is the foolproof way that my mom and I have always made canna-butter in our kitchen. The thing about making a batch of canna-butter is that it's your ticket to infusing any recipe that calls for butter. You can even use vegan butter or almond butter. Infused brownies, cookies, hot dogs (just slap the butter on the bread), or even popcorn can be created with your canna-butter. The downside is that you're not quite sure of the dose of the butter when it comes to cannabinoids per gram. If you need or desire something more exact, purchase an extract, then infuse the butter with that rather than flower. This will give you a more specific guide for dosing.

TOOLS:

Slow cooker

Cheesecloth

Glass storage
  jar or container
  with snap-on lid

INGREDIENTS:

2 cups (4 sticks) butter

Cannabis trim or flower (decarbed);
  3.5 grams is a good starting amount,
  but feel free to experiment

Continued ➤

INSTRUCTIONS:

1. Set the slow cooker on low.

2. Cut up the butter and place it into the cooker.

3. Once the butter is completely melted, place the cannabis into the cooker and stir gently.

4. Cover and let cook for a minimum of 3 hours. The longer you cook it, the more potent it will become.

5. Turn the cooker off and let it cool, but do not allow the butter to harden.

6. Strain the butter through the cheesecloth into a glass container for storage.

BEWARE: This recipe will make your kitchen extremely loud . . . cannabis slang for an incredibly fragrant smell of cannabis.

Do not let the butter harden before you strain it.

VARIATION: The longer you cook this recipe, the more potent it will become. So try to leave it cooking for a full 24 hours for ultimate dankness.

Infused Canna-Oil

VEGAN **Yield**: 16 ounces **Prep time**: 4 hours

Any type of cooking oil, or even blended cooking oils, can be used for this oil infusion. The only oil you can't use is coconut oil, because it will harden at room temperature. (If you want to infuse coconut oil, use the canna-butter recipe.) Remember that your canna-oil will end up with a green color because of the cannabis. Store it in a cool dark place, and it will last for at least 6 months.

INGREDIENTS:
- **6 cups cooking oil (olive, grapeseed, sunflower, peanut, or a mixture)**
- **19 grams decarbed ground cannabis buds**

INSTRUCTIONS:
1. Mix the cooking oil and the decarbed cannabis in the top of a double boiler.

2. Add water to the bottom of the double boiler. Keep the water level too low to touch the upper pot. Cook the oil and the cannabis at a simmer for 3 hours.

3. Stir every 30 minutes.

4. After 3 hours, strain with cheesecloth.

5. Funnel or pour into a jar or bottle.

The OG
Kush Queen Bath Bomb

VEGAN Yield: 2 cups (1 bath bomb)
Prep time: 20 minutes, plus 24 hours to dry

This is our family recipe, the one that started it all for our business. These infused bath bombs will help you find deeper relaxation and improved sleep and will feel like a full-body massage without the price tag. Make them for yourself, or package them up in candy wrappers and give them as gifts.

TOOLS:

Bowls

Whisk

Dropper or baster (optional)

Bath bomb mold or plastic
    ornament (see Tips)

INGREDIENTS:

¾ cup Infused Canna-Oil
    (page 127)

3 teaspoons castor oil

1 tablespoon essential oil
    of your choice (lavender
    and chamomile are my
    favorites)

1 tablespoon water

5 drops food coloring of your
    choice (optional)

½ cup baking soda

¼ cup Epsom salt

¼ cup cornstarch

¼ cup citric acid

INSTRUCTIONS:

1. In a bowl, mix the canna-oil, castor oil, essential oil, water, and food coloring (if using).

2. In a separate bowl, mix the baking soda, Epsom salt, cornstarch, and citric acid.

3. Slowly add the wet ingredients to the dry, whisking gently. Mixing too fast will chemically activate the citric acid, and your bath bombs will have less fizz. Adding the wet ingredients using a dropper or turkey baster helps avoid this.

4. Once the wet and dry ingredients are completely mixed (the texture will be like wet sand), place the mixture into the mold.

5. Let sit for 24 hours to dry, then remove from the mold.

6. Store your bath bombs in a plastic bag or food storage container. (Make sure to label them cannabis bath bombs.)

TIPS: Bath bomb molds are available at craft shops, where you can also find clear plastic globe Christmas tree ornaments, which snap open and closed and make good molds.

VARIATION: Try adding your favorite essential oils and terpenes with your favorite scents.

Brownie Mary
Chocolate Brownies

NUT FREE **Yield:** 12 brownies **Prep time:** 30 minutes

There's nothing more necessary than experiencing a cannabis brownie (this recipe is named for Mary Jane Rathbun). A cannabis brownie is *the* cannabis dessert. This is a 5 mg dose, which should be safe for newcomers. Remember that it's never cool to serve people cannabis products without their knowledge.

TOOLS:

8-by-8-inch baking pan

Parchment paper

Mixing bowls

INGREDIENTS:

Cooking spray

4 ounces semisweet chocolate, chopped

¾ cup all-purpose flour

¼ cup cocoa powder

1 teaspoon salt

10 tablespoons (1¼ sticks) unsalted butter

2 tablespoons Slow Cooker Canna-Butter (page 125)

1¼ cups granulated sugar

2 large eggs

1 tablespoon vanilla extract

INSTRUCTIONS:

1. Preheat the oven to 340°F/171°C. Spray an 8-by-8-inch baking pan with cooking spray, and line it with parchment paper.

2. In a microwave-safe bowl, melt the chopped chocolate in 30-second intervals. Test in between by stirring with a spoon to see whether the chocolate is melted; sometimes it isn't obvious to the eye.

3. In a small bowl, combine the flour, cocoa powder, and salt.

4. In a large bowl, beat the butter, canna-butter, and sugar until light and fluffy, 5 to 7 minutes. Add the eggs and the vanilla extract, and beat for an additional 5 minutes.

5. Beat in the melted chocolate. Gently fold the dry ingredients into the butter/sugar mixture. Don't overmix! You can tell it's ready when you see an absence of flour lumps—you only want to mix until you don't see any.

6. Bake for 18 to 22 minutes.

7. Remove from the oven and let cool.

8. Cut into 12 even squares, or 24 even squares for a microdose serving.

VARIATION: For a fragrant twist, you can replace the water in this recipe with an equal amount of cold brewed tea, rosewater, or orange blossom water. You can also add up to 10 drops of food-grade essential oil if you don't like the hempy taste.

Vegetable Glycerin Tincture

VEGAN **Yield**: 12 ounces **Prep time**: 2 months

Many tinctures are made with alcohol, but I love the gentle nature of this vegetable glycerin tincture. Oil infusions become saturated with cannabinoids and terpenes. Tinctures are the best nonsmokable way to ingest cannabis or infuse it into food or drink. They are perfect for traveling because they are discreet and carry no smell.

TOOLS:

Glass jar with lid

Cheesecloth

Tincture bottle with dropper

Funnel

INGREDIENTS:

7 grams dried decarbed cannabis flower, coarsely ground

12 ounces vegetable glycerin

INSTRUCTIONS:

When making tinctures, the potency of the cannabis will determine the dose. With this recipe, use cannabis with 15 percent THC content. This will mean your tincture is about 5 mg of THC per ½ teaspoon. You may want to use more or less depending on your needs.

1. Place the decarboxylated cannabis in a clean glass jar.

2. Pour the glycerin into the jar, being sure that the glycerin covers the cannabis completely.

3. Secure the jar with an airtight lid and gently mix the contents by rolling the jar back and forth in your hands.

4. Keep the jar in a cool dark place for 2 months. Gently shake the jar every few days.

5. After 2 months, strain out the plant material with cheesecloth. To do this, stretch the cheesecloth across the top of a large spouted measuring cup or bowl and secure it in place with a rubber band or twine.

6. Carefully pour the infused glycerin over the cheesecloth.

7. Lift the cheesecloth and squeeze any remaining glycerin into the cup or bowl. Discard the cheesecloth and solids.

8. Pour the glycerin into a glass jar or tincture bottle, using a funnel. Store in a cool, dark place.

VARIATION: If you don't want to use THC flower, replace it with CBD-dominant flower to make a CBD tincture. If you prefer a flavoring, you can add lavender, peppermint, or your favorite flavor.

Essential Oil Lip Balm

Yield: 2 cups **Prep time**: 15 minutes

A cannabis-infused lip balm will calm and rejuvenate your dry, cracked lips. You'll find yourself endlessly reapplying this lip balm. Customize it with your favorite essential oil. Toss it in your gym bag or makeup bag or take it with you when you travel. This gentle formula won't make you break out, and the cannabis will keep your lips super soft.

TOOLS:

Heatproof glass jar

Cooking thermometer

Lip balm containers (search online, or use small tins or screw-top glass jars or vials)

INGREDIENTS:

1 tablespoon beeswax pellets

3 tablespoons sweet almond oil, avocado oil, or hemp oil

1 tablespoon Infused Canna-Oil (page 127)

15 drops essential oil (try lavender, lemon, or peppermint)

INSTRUCTIONS:

1. Place the beeswax, sweet almond oil, and infused canna-oil in a heatproof glass jar. Fill a saucepan with a couple of inches of water and bring it to a simmer over medium-high heat.

2. Place the jar in the pan. Stir periodically until all the ingredients are fully melted. Turn the heat down if the water begins to boil.

3. Once everything has melted, remove the jar and allow it to cool slightly, until the contents are 140°F/60°C. Add the drops of essential oil and mix well to combine.

4. While the mixture is still liquid, pour it into your desired containers.

Infused Sugar Scrub

Yield: 2 cups **Prep time**: 15 minutes

This refreshing scrub is perfect for dry, cracked skin, although it is not recommended for use on your face. The organic sugar base, CBD, and vitamin E oil will work together to remove dead skin, clean pores, moisturize, and leave your skin glowing. It's great for all skin types and for full-body use, from your elbows to your feet. Fun fact: we have extra-large pores on our feet for absorbing CBD and essential oils.

TOOLS:

Glass mixing bowl

Mason jar with lid

INGREDIENTS:

½ cup coconut oil
  or organic olive oil

¼ cup organic sugarcane

1 teaspoon vitamin E oil

10 drops essential oil
  of your choice

3 grams Infused Canna-Oil
  (page 127)

INSTRUCTIONS:

1. In a glass bowl, mix the coconut oil, sugarcane, vitamin E oil, essential oil, and canna-oil.

2. Massage the mixture together for 5 minutes or until fully incorporated.

3. Transfer to a mason jar or plastic container.

4. Keep near the sink or in the shower for the perfect infused sugar scrub for winter.

Jello Tech Gummy Bears

Yield: 2 cups **Prep time**: 15 minutes

Gummy molds are available from craft stores and specialty cooking stores; any candy-making molds will also work for this recipe. Keep in mind that the fewer/larger molds you use, the higher the dose of each gummy will be. Bite-size is your best bet.

TOOLS:

Microwave-safe bowl

Gummy molds

Spatula

INGREDIENTS:

⅓ cup water

1 box (2 packets) gelatin mix

2.2 grams Infused Canna-Oil (page 127)

INSTRUCTIONS:

1. Place the water in a microwave-safe bowl, add the gelatin, and let it bloom for 5 minutes.

2. Heat the oil in the microwave for 2 minutes or until fully liquefied.

3. Mix the oil into the gelatin.

4. Heat the mixture in the microwave for 1 minute.

5. Pour the mixture into the molds.

6. Use a spatula to smooth and evenly distribute the mixture.

7. Let the mixture cool in the molds until solid.

VARIATION: If you don't have a mold, just pour the mix onto a rimmed baking sheet. Once it solidifies, cut the gelatin into bite-size squares.

Green Machine Smoothie

VEGAN **Yield:** 2½ cups **Prep time**: 15 minutes

We're living in a modern age when cannabis is medicine, so take your dose in this delicious smoothie. One of my favorite ways to enjoy cannabis post workout or to start my day is with this microdosed green machine.

TOOLS:
Blender

Drinking glass or cup

INGREDIENTS:
½ cup kale

1 ripe avocado

1½ cups almond milk

½ cup almond butter

1 teaspoon Slow Cooker Canna-Butter (page 125) or Infused Canna-Oil (page 127)

2 teaspoons hemp or chia seeds

INSTRUCTIONS:
1. In a blender, combine the kale, avocado, almond milk, almond butter, and canna-butter, and process until smooth.

2. Pour into a glass and top with the hemp seeds.

VARIATION: There's so many ways to explore this green machine and make it your own. Add your favorite greens, apples, bananas, or blueberries. You can also add CBD for a perfect ratioed dose.

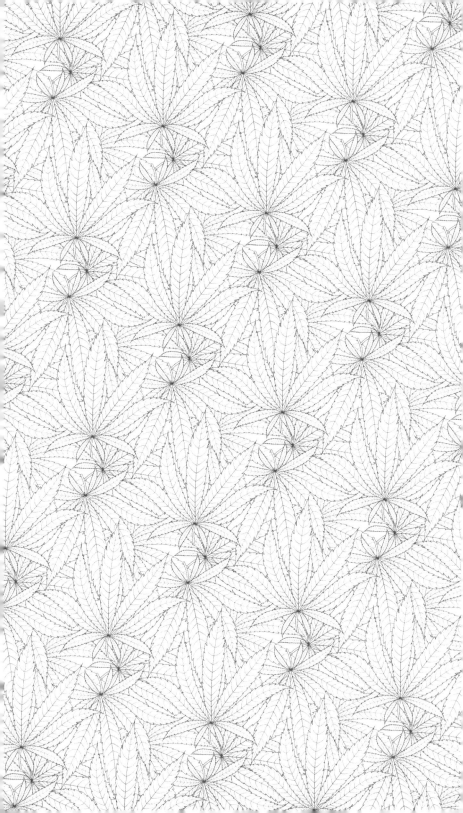

RESOURCES

Education and Databases

Leafly
Cannabis database filled with education, dispensaries, strain information, and growing guides. Leafly.com.

Weed Maps
The industry's oldest dispensary and brand database. WeedMaps.com.

Products and Dispensaries

Columbia Care
Industry leading cannabis and hemp dispensaries. Col-Care.com.

Direct CBD Online
Online marketplace for lab-tested hemp CBD products. DirectCBDOnline.com.

Kush Queen
Handmade, lab-tested, woman-owned since 2015. KushQueen.shop.

Med Men
National cannabis and hemp dispensaries. MedMen.com.

Doctors and Medical Cannabis Care

AIMS Institute
Integrative medical care with real doctors and researchers who know cannabis medicine. AIMSInstitute.net.

American Cannabinoid Clinics
The clinics' mission is "to deliver precision Cannabinoid Medicine to every patient looking for a personalized approach to healing." TheACClinics.com.

Canna-Centers
Medical practice providing patient education on cannabis therapy. Canna-Centers.com.

HelloMD

Online access to doctors, education, and product recommendations. HelloMD.com.

Communities and Support Groups

Endo Black

Pro-cannabis organization dedicated to supporting women with endometriosis. EndoBlack.org.

Cannaclusive

Online community dedicated to fair representation of minorities in cannabis. Cannaclusive.com.

Grief and Cannabis

Cannabis-friendly, wellness-centered grief resources and support. GriefandCannabis.com.

Stoned and Toned

Online fitness and cannabis community. StonedandToned.com.

Addiction and Substance Abuse Support

Beit T'Shuvah

A residential treatment center dedicated to a spiritual and community approach to addiction. BeitTShuvah.org.

Substance Abuse and Mental Health Services Administration Helpline

A national helpline for free, confidential treatment referral information available 24/7, 365 days a year. 1-800-662-HELP(4357). SAMHSA.gov/find-help/national-helpline.

Advocacy, Reform, and Social Justice

Americans for Safe Access

Americans for Safe Access is dedicated to the progress of cannabis as a therapeutic. SafeAccessNow.org.

Drug Policy Alliance

Organization dedicated to ending the war on drugs and prohibtion. DrugPolicy.org.

Last Prisoner Project

An advocacy organization dedicated to cannabis criminal justice reform. LastPrisonerProject.org.

NORML

Organization dedicated to the reform of cannabis policy and advocacy. NORML.org.

REFERENCES

Abioye, Amos et al. "Δ9-Tetrahydrocannabivarin (THCV): A Commentary on Potential Therapeutic Benefit for the Management of Obesity and Diabetes." *Journal of Cannabis Research* 2 (2020): 6. doi.org/10.1186/s42238-020-0016-7.

Abrahamov, Aya et al. "An Efficient New Cannabinoid Antiemetic in Pediatric Oncology." *Life Sciences* 56, no. 23–24 (May 5, 1995): 2097–102. doi.org/10.1016/0024-3205(95)00194-B.

Americans for Safe Access. "Information on Cannabis Safety." Accessed October 6, 2021. SafeAccessNow.org/cannabis_safety.

Anson, Pat. "Harvard Study Finds Cannabis Effective for Chronic Pain." Pain News Network, April 10, 2021. PainNewsNetwork.org/stories/2021/4/10/harvard-study-finds-cannabis-effective-treatment-for-chronic-pain.

Boehnke, Kevin F. et al. "Medical Cannabis Use Is Associated with Decreased Opiate Medication Use in a Retrospective Cross-Sectional Survey of Patients with Chronic Pain." *Journal of Pain* 17, no. 6 (June 1, 2016): 739–44. doi.org/10.1016/j.jpain.2016.03.002.

Brugnatelli, Viola. "Anti-inflammatory and Anti-nociceptive Properties of β-Myrcene." Fundación CANNA. Accessed October 5, 2021. Fundacion-Canna.es/en/anti-inflammatory-anti-nociceptive-properties-v-myrcene.

Cabral, Guy A. et al. "Turning Over a New Leaf: Cannabinoid and Endocannabinoid Modulation of Immune Function." *Journal of Neuroimmune Pharmacology* 10, no. 2 (June 2015): 193–203. doi.org/10.1007/s11481-015-9615-z.

Callaghan, Russell C. et al. "Marijuana Use and Risk of Lung Cancer: A 40-Year Cohort Study." *Cancer Causes and Control* 24, no. 10 (October 2013): 1811–20. doi.org/10.1007/s10552-013-0259-0.

Canna Campus. "Terpenes." March 31, 2019. MyCannaCampus.com/blog /f/terpenes.

Chou, Victor. "The Real Side Effects of Medical Marijuana." January 14, 2019. ChouMD.com/the-real-side-effects-of-medical-marijuana.

Compton, Wilson M. et al. "Medical Marijuana Laws and Cannabis Use: Intersections of Health and Policy." *JAMA Psychiatry* 74, no. 6 (June 2017): 559–60. doi.org/10.1001/jamapsychiatry.2017.0723.

Cuttler, Carrie et al. "A Naturalistic Examination of the Perceived Effects of Cannabis on Negative Affect." *Journal of Affective Disorders* 235 (August 1, 2018): 198–205. doi.org/10.1016/j.jad.2018.04.054.

Dahlhamer, James et al. "Prevalence of Chronic Pain and High-Impact Chronic Pain among Adults—United States, 2016." *Centers for Disease Control and Prevention Morbidity and Mortality Weekly Report* 67, no. 36 (September 14, 2018): 1001–6. doi.org/10.15585/mmwr.mm6736a2.

De Luca, M. A. et al. "Cannabinoid Facilitation of Behavioral and Bio-chemical Hedonic Taste Responses." *Neuropharmacology* 63, no. 1 (July 2012): 161–68. doi.org/10.1016/j.neuropharm.2011.10.018.

Denson, Thomas F., and Mitchell Earleywine. "Decreased Depression in Marijuana Users." *Addictive Behaviors* 31, no. 4 (April 2006): 738–42. doi.org/10.1016/j.addbeh.2005.05.052.

Donahue, Michelle Z. "Earliest Evidence for Cannabis Smoking Dis-covered in Ancient Tombs." *National Geographic*, June 12, 2019. NationalGeographic.com/culture/article/earliest-evidence-cannabis -marijuana-smoking-china-tombs.

Dubovsky, Steven. "Is Cannabis an Analgesic?" *NEJM Journal Watch*, October 5, 2018. JWatch.org/na47647/2018/10/05 /cannabis-analgesic.

Epstein, Jodie. "4 Facts about Cannabis and Migraine That Might Surprise You." Healthline, April 22, 2021. Healthline.com/health/migraine /facts-about-cannabis-and-migraine-that-might-surprise-you.

Fichtner, Christopher G., and Howard B. Moss. "Medical Marijuana and Mental Health: Cannabis Use in Psychiatric Practice." *Psychiatric Times* 34, no. 5 (May 31, 2017). PsychiatricTimes.com/view/medical-marijuana -and-mental-health-cannabis-use-psychiatric-practice.

García, C. et al. "Symptom-Relieving and Neuroprotective Effects of the Phytocannabinoid Δ^9-THCV in Animal Models of Parkinson's Dis-ease." *British Journal of Pharmacology* 163, no. 7 (August 2011): 1495–506. doi.org/10.1111/j.1476-5381.2011.01278.x.

Garland, Rachel. "7 Surprising Facts about Cannabis and Endometriosis." *Green Flower*, July 19, 2020. News.Green-Flower.com/surprising-facts -about-cannabis-and-endometriosis.

Graczyk, Michał et al. "Prospects for the Use of Cannabinoids in Psychiatric Disorders." *Frontiers in Psychiatry* 12 (March 2021): 620073. doi.org/10.3389/fpsyt.2021.620073.

Grinspoon, Peter. "Cannabidiol (CBD)—What We Know and What We Don't." Harvard Health Publishing, September 24, 2021. Health .Harvard.edu/blog/cannabidiol-cbd-what-we-know-and-what-we-dont -2018082414476.

Gupta, Sanjay. "Why I Changed My Mind on Weed." CNN, August 8, 2013. CNN.com/2013/08/08/health/gupta-changed-mind-marijuana /index.html.

Halperin, Alex. "Marijuana: Is It Time to Stop Using a Word with Racist Roots?" *The Guardian*, January 29, 2018. TheGuardian.com/ society/2018/jan/29/marijuana-name-cannabis-racism.

Hansen, Claire et al. "Where Is Marijuana Legal? A Guide to Marijuana Legalization." *U.S. News and World Report*, October 14, 2021. USNews. com/news/best-states/articles/where-is-marijuana-legal-a-guide-to -marijuana-legalization.

Hill, Kevin P. "Medical Marijuana for Treatment of Chronic Pain and Other Medical and Psychiatric Problems: A Clinical Review." *JAMA* 313, no. 24 (June 23/30, 2015): 2474–83. doi.org/10.1001/jama.2015.6199.

Honi Soit. "Harvard Researchers Get High . . . Then Drunk." February 28, 2013. HoniSoit.com/2013/02/harvard-researchers-get-high-then-drunk.

Kassam, Zara. "Cannabinoids Suitable for Migraine Prevention." *European Pharmaceutical Review*, June 29, 2017. EuropeanPharmaceuticalReview. com/news/62784/cannabinoids-suitable-migraine-prevention.

Kennedy, Michael C. "Cannabis: Exercise Performance and Sport: A Systematic Review." *Journal of Science and Medicine in Sport* 20, no. 9 (September 1, 2017): 825–29. doi.org/10.1016/j.jsams.2017.03.012.

Klahn, Philipp. "Cannabinoids—Promising Antimicrobial Drugs or Intoxicants with Benefits?" *Antibiotics* 9, no. 6 (June 2020): 297. doi.org/10.3390/antibiotics9060297.

Kola, Blerina et al. "Cannabinoids and Ghrelin Have Both Central and Peripheral Metabolic and Cardiac Effects via AMP-Activated Protein Kinase." *Journal of Biological Chemistry* 280, no. 26 (July 2005): 25196–201. doi.org/10.1074/jbc.c500175200.

Long, Tengwen et al. "Cannabis in Eurasia: Origin of Human Use and Bronze Age Trans-continental Connections." *Vegetation History and Archaeobotany* 26, no. 2 (March 2017): 245–58. doi.org/10.1007/s00334 -016-0579-6.

Lynn, Becky K. et al. "The Relationship between Marijuana Use Prior to Sex and Sexual Function in Women." *Sexual Medicine* 7, no. 2 (June 1, 2019): 192–97. doi.org/10.1016/j.esxm.2019.01.003.

Margolin, Madison. "Brownie Mary Is the Reason You Can Get Medical Marijuana Today." *Bon Appétit*, April 29, 2019. BonAppetit.com/story /brownie-mary.

McDaniel, Charles et al. "Metals in Cannabis Vaporizer Aerosols: Sources, Possible Mechanisms, and Exposure Profiles." *Chemical Research in Toxicology* 34, no. 11 (November 2021): 2331–42. doi.org/10.1021/acs .chemrestox.1c00230.

Mead, William B. "Mead Says Marijuana Should Be Legalized." *Golden Daily Transcript*, October 27, 1969. ColoradoHistoricNewspapers.org.

Mikolašević, Ivana et al. "Cannabis-Induced Acute Pancreatitis." *Medicinski glasnik: Official Publication of the Medical Association of Zenica-Doboj Canton, Bosnia and Herzegovina* 10, no. 2 (August 2013): 405–7. Ljkzedo.ba/volume-volumen-10-number-broj-2-aug-2013.

Miller, Richard J. *Drugged: The Science and Culture behind Psychotropic Drugs.* New York: Oxford University Press, 2014.

Mullen, Caitlin. "Cannabis Use Is on the Rise among Women: Here's How Their Habits Differ from Men's." *Bizwomen*, June 30, 2021. Bizjournals.com/bizwomen/news/latest-news/2021/06/women-turn -to-cannabis-to-manage-pandemic-anxiety.html.

National Institute on Drug Abuse. "Does Marijuana Use Affect Driving?" April 13, 2021. DrugAbuse.gov/publications/research-reports /marijuana/does-marijuana-use-affect-driving.

National Institute on Drug Abuse. "How Does Marijuana Produce Its Effects?" April 13, 2021. DrugAbuse.gov/publications/research-reports /marijuana/how-does-marijuana-produce-its-effects.

Ngueta, Gerard et al. "Cannabis Use in Relation to Obesity and Insulin Resistance in the Inuit Population." *Obesity* 23, no. 2 (February 2015): 290–95. doi.org/10.1002/oby.20973.

NORML. "Racial Disparity in Marijuana Arrests." Accessed September 29, 2021. NORML.org/marijuana/fact-sheets/racial-disparity-in-marijuana-arrests.

North American Menopause Society. "Cannabis Use for Menopause Symptom Management." September 28, 2020. Menopause.org/docs/default-source/press-release/cannabis-use-for-menopause-9-17-20.pdf.

Popken, Ben. "The Future of Cannabis Is Female: Gen Z Women Are Fastest-Growing Consumers of Legal Weed." NBC News, July 18, 2021. NBCNews.com/business/business-news/future-cannabis-female-gen-z-women-are-fastest-growing-consumers-n1274253.

Powell, Alvin. "What We Know and Don't Know about Pot." *Harvard Gazette*, February 24, 2020. News.Harvard.edu/gazette/story/2020/02/professor-explores-marijuanas-safe-use-and-addiction.

Priest, Ashley. "William Randolph Hearst—Anslinger's Right Hand in Cannabis Prohibition." Veriheal, August 20, 2020. Veriheal.com/blog/william-randolph-hearst-anslingers-right-hand-in-cannabis-prohibition.

Priory Group. "Why Are Stress Levels among Women 50% Higher than Men?" Accessed October 12, 2021. PrioryGroup.com/blog/why-are-stress-levels-among-women-50-higher-than-men.

Ren, Meng et al. "The Origins of Cannabis Smoking: Chemical Residue Evidence from the First Millennium BCE in the Pamirs." *Science Advances* 5, no. 6 (June 12, 2019): eaaw1391. doi.org/10.1126/sciadv.aaw1391.

Reynolds, Gretchen. "Getting to the Bottom of the Runner's High." *New York Times*, March 10, 2021. NYTimes.com/2021/03/10/well/move/running-exercise-mental-effects.html.

Rhyne, Danielle N. et al. "Effects of Medical Marijuana on Migraine Headache Frequency in an Adult Population." *Pharmacotherapy* 36, no. 5 (May 2016): 505–10. doi.org/10.1002/phar.1673.

Rosenthal, Franz. *The Herb: Hashish versus Medieval Muslim Society*. Leiden: E. J. Brill, 1971.

Schaeffer, Katherine. "6 Facts about Americans and Marijuana." Pew Research Center, April 26, 2021. PewResearch.org/fact-tank/2021/04/26/facts-about-marijuana.

Schafer, Gráinne et al. "Investigating the Interaction between Schizotypy, Divergent Thinking and Cannabis Use." *Consciousness and Cognition* 21, no. 1 (March 2012): 292–98. doi.org/10.1016/j.concog.2011.11.009.

Schaneman, Bart. "Edibles Outperform Cannabis Industry Growth in 2020 on COVID-Spurred Sales Surge." *MJBizDaily*, January 11, 2021. MJBizDaily.com/edibles-outperform-cannabis-industry-growth-in-2020-on-covid-spurred-sales-surge.

Schultz, Rachael. "The Best Ways to Work Weed into Your Workout." *Men's Journal.* Accessed December 13, 2021. MensJournal.com/health-fitness/how-to-work-weed-into-your-workout-thc-cbd-for-recovery.

Simon, Mallory, and Melissa Dunst Lipman. "Charlotte Figi, the Girl Who Inspired a CBD Movement, Has Died at Age 13." CNN, April 9, 2020. CNN.com/2020/04/08/health/charlotte-figi-cbd-marijuana-dies/index.html.

Soria-Gómez, Edgar et al. "The Endocannabinoid System Controls Food Intake via Olfactory Processes." *Nature Neuroscience* 17 (March 2014): 407–15. doi.org/10.1038/nn.3647.

Substance Abuse and Mental Health Services Administration, U.S. Department of Health and Human Services. "Drug Abuse Warning Network (DAWN)." Accessed December 13, 2021. SAMHSA.gov/data/data-we-collect/dawn-drug-abuse-warning-network.

Sun, Andrew J., and Michael L. Eisenberg. "Association between Marijuana Use and Sexual Frequency in the United States: A Population-Based Study." *Journal of Sexual Medicine* 14, no. 11 (November 1, 2017): 1342–47. doi.org/10.1016/j.jsxm.2017.09.005.

Sutherland, Stephani. "Marijuana May Boost, Rather than Dull, the Elderly Brain." *Scientific American*, May 10, 2017. ScientificAmerican.com/article/marijuana-may-boost-rather-than-dull-the-elderly-brain.

Takahashi, R. N., and I. G. Karniol. "Pharmacologic Interaction between Cannabinol and δ^9-Tetrahydrocannabinol." *Psychopharmacologia* 41, no. 3 (January 1975): 277–84. doi.org/10.1007/BF00428937.

Toklas, Alice B. *The Alice B. Toklas Cook Book*. London: Michael Joseph, 1954.

University of Bonn. "Cannabis Reverses Aging Processes in the Brain, Study Suggests: Researchers Restore the Memory Performance of Methuselah Mice to a Juvenile Stage." Science Daily, May 8, 2017. ScienceDaily.com /releases/2017/05/ 170508112400.htm.

U.S. Food and Drug Administration. "FDA Approves First Drug Comprised of an Active Ingredient Derived from Marijuana to Treat Rare, Severe Forms of Epilepsy." June 25, 2018. FDA.gov/news-events /press-announcements/fda-approves-first-drug-comprised-active -ingredient-derived-marijuana-treat-rare-severe-forms.

Vandergriendt, Carly. "Can Medical Marijuana Alleviate Fibromyalgia Symptoms?" Healthline, March 10, 2021. Healthline.com/health /fibromyalgia/marijuana-fibromyalgia.

Vučković, Sonja et al. "Cannabinoids and Pain: New Insights from Old Molecules." *Frontiers in Pharmacology* 9 (November 2018): 1259. doi.org/10.3389/fphar.2018.01259.

Weizman, Libat et al. "Cannabis Analgesia in Chronic Neuropathic Pain Is Associated with Altered Brain Connectivity." *Neurology* 91, no. 14 (October 2, 2018): e1285–e1294. doi.org/10.1212/WNL.0000000000006293.

Wilcox, Anna. "Cannabis for Creativity and Problem Solving? Here's How . . ." Green Flower, July 19, 2020. News.Green-Flower.com /cannabis-and-creativity.

Wilson, Elizabeth B. "The Queen Who Would Be King." *Smithsonian*, September 2006. SmithsonianMag.com/history/the-queen-who -would-be-king-130328511.

INDEX

P

Pain management, 31,
34, 77–79, 85
frequently asked
questions, 83–84
during sex, 105
tips, 81–82
what to use, 79–81
Paranoia, 54
Pepper, for bad
highs, 63
Peron, Dennis, 6
Pharmacological
determinism, 26
Pinene, 13
Playlist, 61
PMS, 32
Potency, 122
Proposition 215 (1996),
4, 69
Proposition P (1991), 6
Pure Food and Drug
Act (1906), 3–4

R

Randall, Robert, 4
Rathbun, Mary Jane, 6, 130
Ratios, 45, 115
Reagan, Ronald, 4
Recipes
Brownie Mary Chocolate
Brownies, 130–131
Essential Oil Lip
Balm, 134
Green Machine Smoothie, 137
Infused Canna-Oil, 127
Infused Sugar Scrub, 135
Jello Tech Gummy
Bears, 136

The OG Kush Queen Bath
Bomb, 128–129
Slow Cooker Canna-
Butter, 125–126
Vegetable Glycerin
Tincture, 132–133
Reefer Madness (film), 4
Runner's high, 55, 95–96, 101
Ryan, Sophie, 28

S

Safety guidelines, 23–24
San Francisco Cannabis
Buyers Club, 6
Sativa strains, 15–16
Sexual health, 33, 102–103,
110, 115, 118
frequently asked
questions, 108–109
tips, 106–107
what to use, 104, 105–106
Side effects, 23–24
Skin conditions, 33, 92, 93, 94.
See also Beauty products,
cannabis-infused
Sleep, 34, 35, 74,
102–103, 110, 115
frequently asked
questions, 108
tips, 106–107
what to use, 103–104
Slow Cooker Canna-
Butter, 125–126
Smoking, 18–19, 58
Smoothie, Green
Machine, 137
Strains, 14–17
Stress relief, 31–32, 70
Sugar Scrub, Infused, 135

Acknowledgments

I would like to express my deepest gratitude to Michael Sawyer, who has taught me everything I know about the science of cannabis. I would like to thank Tiffany Whitmore, for believing in me as a writer and content creator. To my Kush Queen team, who suffer my daily complaints and always commit to bringing cannabis wellness to the masses, every single day. I couldn't have completed this book without you.

To all the women in cannabis who came before me so I could exist, thank you.

Lastly, cannabis, I love you. You are my medicine and my best friend, and words could never ever capture what you have given me. Thank you for your innate wisdom and healing. It's all because of you.

About the Author

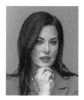

Olivia Alexander is the CEO and founder of Kush Queen and has spent 15 years in the cannabis trenches working to change the face of the cannabis business for the better. By focusing on CBD-infused products and continually improving formulas designed to work with the feminine body, Kush Queen has become one of the most respected and sought-after cannabis wellness brands on the market. The company's combination of game-changing nanotechnology and advanced minor cannabinoid formulas, along with her fun, educational approach to cannabis, has earned Olivia the title "The Mariah Carey of Weed" from *Elle* magazine. She has over one billion impressions as a social media influencer, sharing her own mental health and alternative medicine journey on Instagram and TikTok.